Stroke Recovery

Reclaiming Independence After Stroke

(*A Comprehensive Guide To Holistic Exercises, Rehabilitation, And Support For Rebuilding Overall Health And Well-being)*

Ricardo Allison

Published By **Ryan Princeton**

Ricardo Allison

All Rights Reserved

Stroke Recovery: Reclaiming Independence After Stroke (A Comprehensive Guide To Holistic Exercises, Rehabilitation, And Support For Rebuilding Overall Health And Well-being)

ISBN 978-1-7773611-0-5

No part of this guidebook shall be reproduced in any form without permission in writing from the publisher except in the case of brief quotations embodied in critical articles or reviews.

Legal & Disclaimer

The information contained in this book is not designed to replace or take the place of any form of medicine or professional medical advice. The information in this book has been provided for educational & entertainment purposes only.

The information contained in this book has been compiled from sources deemed reliable, and it is accurate to the best of the Author's knowledge; however, the Author cannot guarantee its accuracy and validity and cannot be held liable for any errors or omissions. Changes are periodically made to this book. You must consult your doctor or get professional medical advice before using any of the suggested remedies, techniques, or information in this book.

Upon using the information contained in this book, you agree to hold harmless the Author from and against any damages, costs, and expenses, including any legal fees potentially resulting from the application of any of the information provided by this guide. This disclaimer applies to any damages or injury caused by the use and application, whether directly or indirectly, of any advice or information presented, whether for breach of contract, tort, negligence, personal injury, criminal intent, or under any other cause of action.

You agree to accept all risks of using the information presented inside this book. You need to consult a professional medical practitioner in order to ensure you are both able and healthy enough to participate in this program.

Table Of Contents

Chapter 1: The Stroke Journey 1

Chapter 2: Affects Mental, Personal, And Emotional Functions 16

Chapter 3: Hospitalization And Urgent Care 24

Chapter 4: Overcoming Early Emotional And Physical Difficulties 33

Chapter 5: Occupational Therapy For Personal Suitability 46

Chapter 6: Emotional Assimilations And Coping Methods...................................... 63

Chapter 7: Adaptive Equipment And Mobility Assistants.................................. 76

Chapter 8: Technology That Is Accessible For Independent Living 91

Chapter 9: Sleep And Renewal Activities 105

Chapter 10: Management Of Cholesterol And Blood Pressure............................. 118

Chapter 11: The Many Movements Of The Shoulder Joint 132

Chapter 12: Transverse Abdominal Muscle 149

Chapter 13: The Chest Muscles 166

Chapter 14: The Non-Affected Hand 181

Chapter 1: The Stroke Journey

The enjoy of getting a stroke is deep and existence-converting, and it has a big impact on each the individual that has it and their loved ones The signs and symptoms and symptoms of a stroke appear all of sudden and might exchange depending on the a part of the thoughts this is damaged. Sudden numbness or weakening of the face, arm, or leg, usually on one factor of the body, hassle speaking or statistics speech, a severe headache, vertigo, loss of coordination or stability, and imaginative and prescient issues are a number of the common signs and symptoms and signs and symptoms. It is critical to are searching for for clinical help right away if these signs and symptoms and signs and symptoms appear due to the reality activate motion can extensively enhance results and reduce lengthy-time period problems.

When stroke patients arrive on the health center, a multidisciplinary organization of medical professionals with facts in stroke care brief assesses them. Together, those committed human beings stabilize the affected character, decide the sort and basis of the stroke, and begin the critical remedies. Time is of the essence considering the fact that a few treatments, together with mechanical clot extraction or thrombolytic remedy, paintings first-rate when administered inside a particular window of time after the onset of signs.

A stroke survivor is a monument to the tenacity and fortitude of the human spirit. But the road to healing is often prolonged and hard. Depending at the stroke's severity, someone might also enjoy bodily, intellectual, and emotional worrying conditions that call for enormous remedy and assistance.

Strength, coordination, and motor talents are all desires of physical remedy. To cope with unique deficits, it may require severa treatments, which includes physiotherapy, occupational treatment, and speech remedy.

These instructions deal with growing mobility and balance average, relearning speech and language abilities, and enhancing independence in daily obligations.

Another critical step within the restoration technique after a stroke is cognitive rehabilitation. Cognitive troubles, collectively with reminiscence loss, interest troubles, annoying conditions with trouble-solving, or abnormalities in belief, may also occur in brilliant stroke survivors. Cognitive remedy assists sufferers in regaining cognitive functioning, adjusting to novel situations, and growing coping mechanisms.

Both stroke survivors and their carers gain notably from emotional useful useful resource for the duration of the recuperation device. The emotional toll of a stroke may be excessive and consist of feelings like worry, rage, sadness, frustration, or even depression. A revel in of community and information can be created via beneficial useful resource businesses, remedy, and interaction with wonderful stroke survivors. These sports moreover offer people a dialogue board to talk about their studies, insights, and coping techniques.

Stroke survivors frequently must modify their lifestyles to decrease their threat of having a few different stroke, further to dealing with the physical and emotional results. A healthful diet, regular workout, stress control, stopping smoking, and precise manipulate of underlying illnesses which embody excessive blood strain, diabetes, and excessive ldl ldl cholesterol are some examples of those adjustments.

The adventure following a stroke impacts no longer actually the person that had it, however moreover their cherished ones. Family contributors and extraordinary caregivers are especially vital in supplying help, concept, and assist in the end of the healing manner. They can need to change their life to deal with logo-new problems, maintain a solid surroundings, and assist with every day responsibilities.

Despite the large barriers that a stroke affords, many humans float directly to reconstruct their lives and discover sparkling which means that and desires. Resilience, personal development, and a renewed appreciation for lifestyles's easy pleasures are frequently fostered thru the stroke experience. Stroke survivors can reclaim their freedom, feel empowered yet again, and assemble worthwhile futures with the resource of embracing rehabilitation, seeking out assist, and maintaining a first-rate outlook.

The stroke adventure serves as a reminder of the notable power of the human spirit to endure worry. It demonstrates the charge of elevating popularity approximately stroke, taking steps to save you it, and doing ongoing research to beautify available remedies.

STROKE TYPES AND CAUSES

A stroke is a scientific sickness wherein mind cells die due to faded or interrupted blood supply to the mind. There are severa stroke sorts, and each has its specific reasons and tendencies. Ischemic stroke, hemorrhagic stroke, and transient ischemic assault (TIA) are the three crucial types of stroke. Let's examine every type in extra element:

Ischemic Stroke: Ischemic strokes, which make up spherical eighty% of all strokes, appear whilst a blood artery that substances the mind is blocked or constricts, reducing blood drift. Ischemic stroke can rise up in precise subtypes:

a. Thrombotic Stroke: A blood clot paperwork in one of the arteries that deliver blood to the mind, ensuing in this kind of stroke. The clot generally paperwork wherein atherosclerosis, a ailment marked through manner of the accumulation of fatty deposits (plaque) in the arteries, has already taken vicinity.

b. Embolic Stroke: An embolic stroke takes location whilst a blood clot or exclusive piece of particles develops some other place in the frame, regularly in the coronary heart, and moves through the bloodstream until it blocks a smaller artery within the brain.

Hemorrhagic Stroke: About 20% of all strokes are hemorrhagic strokes, which arise whilst a blood artery inside the mind bursts, ensuing in bleeding into or across the thoughts. Hemorrhagic stroke may be of two vital sorts:

a. Intracerebral Hemorrhage: When a blood vessel inside the mind bursts, bleeding within the mind tissue effects. Intracerebral bleeding regularly results from cerebral amyloid angiopathy and excessive blood stress.

b. A subarachnoid hemorrhage is characterized via the usage of the use of bleeding inside the location the various mind and the sensitive tissues covering it. It often consequences from the rupture of an arteriovenous malformation (AVM) or an aneurysm (a vulnerable, bulging blood vessel) in the mind.

A brief ischemic assault, additionally known as a "mini-stroke," is a brief disruption of blood go with the flow to the thoughts. It happens due to a temporary blockage or clot. TIAs commonly simplest very last a couple of minutes and do not harm the thoughts actually. They have to be dealt with significantly because of the fact they may be signs of a destiny stroke.

Risk Factors: A few subjects ought to make you more likely to have a stroke. These embody:

a. The fundamental risk element for stroke is excessive blood strain (excessive blood pressure).

b. Smoking: Smoking reasons blood vessels to visit pot and increases the risk of blood clots.

c. Diabetes: Blood vessel harm and an extended chance of atherosclerosis are each because of excessive blood sugar ranges.

d. High Cholesterol: The production of plaque can be aided via using manner of progressed tiers of LDL (horrible) cholesterol.

e. Atrial Fibrillation: An ordinary heartbeat with a view to growth the risk of growing blood clots within the coronary coronary coronary heart that spread to the mind.

f. Obesity and Physical Inactivity: Having a sedentary manner of existence and being overweight each increase the hazard of stroke.

g. Alcohol Abuse: Drinking excessive portions of alcohol can enhance blood stress and boom the danger of hemorrhagic stroke.

h. Family facts: The hazard is extended with the useful resource of getting a close to family who has experienced a stroke.

i. Age and Gender: Stroke hazard rises with advancing age, and men generally have a bigger risk than premenopausal girls.

j. The danger of stroke may be extended thru way of numerous medical situations, along side coronary coronary coronary heart contamination, sickle cell ailment, and autoimmune illnesses.

It's essential to be conscious that strokes also can be divided into companies based on in which they upward thrust up within the thoughts, along side anterior circulation strokes, which have an effect at the the front segment of the thoughts, and posterior circulate strokes, that have an effect at the again. Additionally, strokes may be in addition divided primarily based at the etiology, together with lacunar stroke (due to tiny vessel ailment) or cardioembolic stroke (due to a clot coming from the coronary coronary heart).

Every shape of stroke desires fast scientific interest because of the reality the mind desires oxygen and nutrients to feature nicely continuously. Rapid assessment and treatment are critical to reducing mind damage and improving recovery possibilities. Call emergency offerings right away in case you or a person close by well-known signs and symptoms of a stroke, which includes abrupt weakness, numbness, problem talking, excruciating headache, or lack of coordination.

STROKE: IMMEDIATE MEDICAL ACTION

A stroke need to be dealt with medically as short as viable to reduce thoughts damage and increase healing potentialities. A stroke, frequently referred to as a cerebrovascular accident (CVA), occurs on the equal time because the thoughts's blood deliver is cut off, every because of a blocked blood artery (ischemic stroke) or thoughts hemorrhage (hemorrhagic stroke). When it involves stroke, time is the vital detail because of the reality the thoughts cells can begin to die truely minutes after the stroke begins offevolved offevolved. The protection of thoughts function thru short clinical hobby can help keep away from everlasting incapacity or possibly demise. The instant medical response to a stroke is printed in detail here:

Understanding the signs and symptoms is the primary level within the preliminary clinical reaction to a stroke. Sudden susceptible factor or numbness on one thing of the face, arm, or leg, confusion, difficulty speaking or expertise, problem walking, lack of stability or coordination, a excessive headache, and blurred or double vision are all not unusual signs and symptoms and signs and symptoms and symptoms of a stroke. People want to be privy to those signs and symptoms and take them critically, every for themselves and for the humans spherical them.

Emergency scientific services (EMS) activation: It's crucial to dial emergency services right away if someone famous stroke symptoms and symptoms. The emergency quantity is 911 in numerous nations. By calling EMS, you may ensure that professional medical employees will arrive without delay and supply the care you want.

Rapid exam and transportation: EMS human beings will examine the affected man or woman's scenario and take a brief medical data even as they arrive. To determine the severity of the stroke, they may degree important symptoms such as blood pressure, coronary coronary coronary heart charge, and oxygen ranges as well as conduct a neurological examination. They will make preparations for set off transportation to the closest stroke middle or sanatorium with stroke capabilities primarily based on their findings and administer the right remedy.

Pre-hospital notification: To alert the receiving clinic of important statistics on the affected man or woman's popularity, EMS frame of employees will also get in contact with them. This pre-clinic alert assists the health center in being prepared for the advent of the stroke affected character, allowing a quick and powerful reaction.

Transport to a stroke middle: Stroke patients need to, each time viable, be taken to a hospital or particular stroke center that gives professional stroke care. These hospitals encompass agencies specifically targeted on treating stroke patients, on the side of neurologists, neurosurgeons, and knowledgeable stroke nurses. Advanced imaging system, at the side of computed tomography (CT) and magnetic resonance imaging (MRI), are to be had at stroke centers to aid in the analysis of the sort and vicinity of strokes.

Administration of time-sensitive remedies: Time-touchy treatments may be began as brief as feasible, relying on the sort and severity of the stroke. The wonderful treatment for ischemic strokes, which make up the majority of strokes, is the early intravenous infusion of tissue plasminogen activator (tPA). By dissolving the blood clot that's inflicting the stroke, this clot-busting drug can assist the broken a part of the thoughts get its blood float once more. Endovascular remedy, which makes use of catheters and stents to physical eliminate or break up the clot, additionally may be applied in a few situations.

Supportive care: Stroke patients want supportive care similarly to drug remedies that want to be administered rapid to assist them control their signs and symptoms and signs and avoid complications. This can entail administering oxygen, controlling blood pressure, and the use of capsules to prevent seizures, reduce mind swelling, and control wonderful clinical issues. To offer them with steady supervision and the vital care, stroke patients are regularly admitted to an intensive care unit or a devoted stroke unit.

Rehabilitation and healing: Following the crowning glory of urgent scientific treatment for a stroke, attention turns to rehabilitation and recuperation. Physical remedy, occupational therapy, speech and language treatment, and mental help are all included in a whole stroke rehabilitation application.

Chapter 2: Affects Mental, Personal, And Emotional Functions

A character's bodily, cognitive, and emotional abilties can all be considerably impacted via a stroke.

Physical Activities:

Hemiparesis, additionally known as hemiplegia, is the weakening or paralysis of one aspect of the frame introduced on thru a stroke. The potential to stroll, perform each day tasks, and manipulate motions may be impacted with the aid of this.

Sensation: Sensory abnormalities added on by way of manner of a stroke may additionally moreover embody numbness or loss of sensation on one difficulty of the body. Proprioception (interest of bodily function) and the senses of touch, temperature, and ache can be impacted by means of the use of this.

Stroke survivors may moreover war with stability and coordination, that would make it difficult for them to walk and preserve stability.

Speech and Swallowing: A situation called dysphagia takes place whilst people have trouble producing speech, expertise language, and swallowing. This is relying on the place and severity of the stroke.

Cognitive Processes

Stroke can have an effect on reminiscence capabilities, which includes quick-time period reminiscence and the functionality to recall contemporary events. Additionally, it is able to affect interest span, making it hard to attention and pay attention to responsibilities.

Language and Communication: A commonplace cognitive side effect of stroke is aphasia, a language hassle. It also can moreover result in issues with writing, reading, talking, and records language.

Executive Functions: Problem-fixing, decision-making, making plans, and organizational competencies are the numerous govt competencies that is probably impacted via a stroke. The sports of every day dwelling and social relationships can be impacted via the usage of those limitations.

Emotional competencies: Depression and tension are feasible emotional changes that stroke patients might also enjoy. The physical guidelines and cognitive adjustments delivered on with the beneficial aid of the stroke can also make a contribution to these emotional troubles.

Emotional Liability: Some people are vulnerable to emotional lability, it truly is characterized with the resource of the usage of abrupt mood adjustments, uncontrollable crying or giggling, or overly emotional reactions.

Stroke must have an effect on someone's self-esteem and capacity to address the troubles of rehabilitation. A loss of self warranty, issue adjusting to the new regular, and frustration are viable effects of the modifications in bodily and cognitive capacities.

It is big to awareness on that a stroke's outcomes can variety from individual to man or woman relying at the amount and region of the damage to the mind. Physical treatment, occupational treatment, speech remedy, and intellectual counseling are all important additives of rehabilitation packages that useful useful resource stroke survivors in regaining function and elevating their great of existence.

THE NEED FOR REHABILITATION

For stroke survivors to heal and maintain their prolonged-time period well-being, stroke rehabilitation is essential. A stroke need to have extreme aftereffects, which consist of physical, intellectual, and emotional troubles. Stroke survivors can, but, repair misplaced talents, enhance their splendid of existence, and reintegrate into their normal sports activities with activate and green rehabilitation.

Restoring Physical Function: Restoring bodily function is one of the maximum crucial desires of stroke recovery. Individuals may additionally moreover have weakness or paralysis on one aspect of the body, problems with balance and coordination, or decreased mobility, relying on the vicinity of the thoughts damaged through the stroke. These issues are addressed by way of rehabilitation techniques like physical remedy, occupational treatment, and speech treatment. Therapists assist stroke sufferers to repair energy, growth variety of movement, improve coordination and relearn necessary capabilities like strolling, eating, dressing, and talking via tailored carrying occasions. The bodily characteristic need to be recovered to regain independence and carry out each day chores.

Enhancing Cognitive Abilities: Strokes also can bring about cognitive deficits, which limit someone's potential to do not forget topics, pay hobby, clear up issues, and communicate. These problems are addressed thru rehabilitation strategies like cognitive remedy and neuropsychological opinions. Individuals can decorate their cognitive skills, trap up on any closing deficiencies, and get better best cognitive functioning thru carrying out cognitive sports activities sports. Cognitive rehabilitation permits stroke survivors complete obligations greater effectively even as moreover boosting their shallowness and popular highbrow health.

Addressing Emotional and Psychological Needs: Stroke rehabilitation is aware of how the stroke has affected the survivors and their cherished one's feelings and mental nicely-being. Anxiety, despair, dissatisfaction, and a dwindled revel in of self-worth may give up end result from the abrupt lack of independence, manner of existence adjustments, and rehabilitation problems. Rehabilitation applications often contain counseling, resource businesses, and mental assist to resource sufferers and their households in overcoming those emotional problems. It is crucial for stroke survivors' typical healing and variation to lifestyles after the stroke to attend to their emotional desires.

Preventing Secondary outcomes: Muscle contractures, stress sores, urinary tract infections, and pneumonia are most of the secondary effects that stroke survivors are much more likely to have. Preventive techniques are included into rehabilitation packages to reduce the chance of these issues. For example, occupational therapists can provide advice on positioning and strain comfort techniques, bodily therapists can train stroke survivors wearing occasions to maintain muscle energy and joint flexibility, and speech therapists can assist with enhancing swallowing function to lower the threat of aspiration pneumonia. The purpose of stroke rehabilitation is to enhance health consequences and prevent extra health troubles via addressing these functionality repercussions.

Promoting Long-Term Recovery: Rehabilitation following a stroke includes no longer only the without delay healing period but additionally the prolonged-term recuperation way. As they reintegrate into their houses, organizations, and workplaces, stroke survivors often face ongoing issues. Rehabilitation applications help human beings regulate to these modifications through supporting them set practical dreams and teaching them the way to deal with failures. The purpose is to encourage prolonged-time period recovery in order that stroke sufferers can stay fun lives and reap their entire

Chapter 3: Hospitalization And Urgent Care

To reduce harm and useful aid in restoration after a stroke, it's essential to give quick medical hobby to the affected character. To efficiently control stroke sufferers inside the early stages of their restoration technique, acute remedy, and hospitalization are crucial. Stabilizing the affected man or woman, figuring out the sort and severity of the stroke, stopping complications, and starting the proper remedies are normal responsibilities for this degree.

When a stroke incidence occurs, step one in presenting acute care is to name emergency services. The scientific personnel conducts a quick evaluation of the patient as quickly as they get to the sanatorium to gauge their circumstance and understand the shape of stroke they have got had. This assessment often includes a evaluation of the affected person's medical data, physical exams, imaging exams (like CT or MRI scans), and laboratory exams.

Hospitalization in specialised stroke devices or neurology wards is mostly a defining feature of the early stages of stroke restoration. These hospitals have the important device to provide complete care, and people devices are staffed with clinical employees skilled in dealing with stroke sufferers. Hospitalization within the direction of this time has a number of targets, a number of which might be as follows:

Monitoring and stabilization: Stroke sufferers need to have their critical signs and symptoms and signs and signs, which incorporates blood strain, coronary heart charge, and oxygen levels, carefully monitored. To maintain those parameters and save you destiny harm, drugs can be given.

Thrombolysis or mechanical thrombectomy: To reestablish blood flow to the thoughts in some ischemic stroke instances, clot-dissolving drugs (thrombolysis) or mechanical clot elimination (thrombectomy) may be used internal a specific time body. These remedies are meant to lessen the severity of mind damage.

Complications which incorporates pneumonia, deep vein thrombosis, urinary tract infections, and pressure sores are much more likely to get up in stroke sufferers. Hospitalization permits preventative interventions together with early movement, posture, respiration aid, and suitable tablets to restrict those troubles.

Launching rehabilitation treatment options: Launching rehabilitation interventions to resource beneficial recuperation is a crucial a part of early-diploma stroke healing. This have to involve interventions like physical remedy, occupational remedy, speech remedy, and others which are catered to the patient's precise desires. The desires of rehabilitation are to regain misplaced abilties, boom mobility, decorate conversation, and reclaim independence.

Support and emotional treatment are vital for stroke sufferers because of the fact they typically enjoy emotional distress from unanticipated life-converting activities like anxiety, melancholy, or frustration. During hospitalization, clinical personnel can supply sufferers and their households emotional beneficial aid, counseling, and education.

A numerous group of healthcare experts works collectively to ensure complete care all through the intense care and hospitalization stages. Neurologists, stroke professionals, nurses, bodily and occupational therapists, speech therapists, nutritionists, social personnel, and psychologists may also want to all be part of this crew. Regular evaluations are completed to song the affected individual's development, modify treatments, and create custom designed care plans.

After receiving acute care and being admitted to the sanatorium, stroke sufferers can keep their rehabilitation in rehab facilities, professional nursing homes, or thru outpatient rehabilitation applications. The severity of the stroke and the patient's development decide the period and diploma of rehabilitation.

In the early levels of stroke restoration, acute care and hospitalization are important for stabilizing the affected man or woman, figuring out the form of stroke, averting headaches, and beginning the right remedies. During the ones ranges, it is possible to keep a watch constant fixed at the affected man or woman's health, carry out any crucial remedies, and start the rehabilitation technique. Optimizing healing, decreasing impairments, and enhancing affected person quality of life are the principle goals.

MANAGING MEDICAL PROCEDURES AND MEDICATIONS

Stroke healing can be a tough manner requiring cautious manipulate of medication and clinical strategies. Early stroke restoration is crucial for making sure the first rate viable restore and decreasing the opportunity of extra issues. This difficulty seeks to offer thorough insights about administering tablets and gift system scientific strategies eventually of this crucial stage, highlighting the significance of operating with healthcare specialists and following encouraged remedy programs.

Managing medicinal drug:

1. Consultation with Medical Personnel:

It is critical to talk with scientific professionals after a stroke diagnosis, which includes neurologists, physiatrists, and pharmacists, to understand the prescriptions made for stroke rehabilitation.

To make sure thorough statistics and adherence, bypass over each remedy's purpose, dosage, feasible unfavorable outcomes, and interactions.

For the satisfactory advice, address any lingering questions or problems you may have regarding the medicine.

2. Medicine Compliance:

Maintaining adherence to the encouraged drug agenda is critical for handling stroke restoration efficiently.

Plan your every day medication ordinary, which includes dosage times, and employ alarms or reminders to make sure you take your medicinal capsules on time.

Create a time table and encompass taking medicinal tablets in every day sports.

Promptly alert medical personnel to any troubles or bad effects.

3. Types of medicinal tablets:

Antiplatelet Drugs: To save you blood clots and further strokes, docs can also offer capsules like aspirin, clopidogrel, or dipyridamole.

Anticoagulants: Warfarin or unique direct oral anticoagulants (DOACs) can be required at the identical time as atrial stressful infection or different factors that boom the danger of blood clot formation are gift.

Statins: By decreasing levels of cholesterol and decreasing the chance of recurrent stroke, those capsules help.

Blood Pressure Medicine: Reducing excessive blood strain is vital to avoid in addition strokes. You might be given a prescription for drugs like ACE inhibitors, diuretics, or beta-blockers.

Additional Drugs: Additional drugs like antidepressants, muscle relaxants, or anticonvulsants may be administered based on a affected individual's desires and any specific stroke-associated troubles.

Medical Techniques:

1. Diagnostic Techniques:

Healthcare professionals may additionally moreover perform numerous diagnostic techniques at some stage in the initial degrees of stroke recuperation to evaluate the degree of injury and direct remedy choices.

These techniques would possibly in all likelihood encompass echocardiography, electrocardiography (ECG), carotid ultrasonography, or angiography similarly to mind imaging studies (CT take a look at, MRI).

Follow the steering, scheduling, and any dietary or pharmaceutical boundaries advocated through healthcare experts for those processes.

2. Interventions in Rehabilitation:

Rehabilitation is vital to a stroke survivor's rehabilitation. Regaining misplaced capabilities and improving the quality of lifestyles may be helped thru specialised interventions together with physical remedy, occupational treatment, speech therapy, and others.

Chapter 4: Overcoming Early Emotional And Physical Difficulties

A stroke is an surprising, notably changing prevalence which can result in plenty of physical and intellectual problems. However, it is feasible to conquer those preliminary challenges and begin down the street to restoration with the right expertise, guide, and proactive efforts. This article tries to teach readers at the bodily and mental troubles that would get up at a few diploma within the initial levels of stroke restoration and to provide coping mechanisms.

Physical Difficulties:

Muscle weakness or paralysis is one of the most time-venerated physical problems following a stroke. Different regions of the frame can be impacted depending on the part of the mind that is damaged by way of way of the stroke. This may want to make normal things like on foot or deciding on up gadgets quite hard.

Physical therapy: Attending classes would possibly probably help you get stronger and extra cellular. A specialized schooling plan might be created thru an authorized therapist to often beautify muscle feature and increase the range of motion.

Using assistive devices, which includes canes, walkers, or braces, can provide stability and manual in the course of the initial stages of recuperation. These tools assist independence, stability renovation, and fall prevention.

Communication and Speech Issues: Stroke sufferers can also additionally moreover have problem speakme, decoding language, or efficiently expressing themselves. Aphasia is a scenario that may reason isolation and dissatisfaction.

Speech treatment: Relearning verbal exchange talents can be helped thru speech and language remedy. Exercises for word retrieval, language comprehension, and articulation may be furnished with the aid of using a speech therapist.

Alternative verbal exchange strategies: For human beings with excessive aphasia, the use of gestures, writing, or augmentative and opportunity conversation (AAC) gadgets as an alternative to speech can on occasion be beneficial.

Fatigue and Energy Conservation: The physical needs of rehabilitation coupled with the mind's attempts to restoration itself regularly bring about fatigue within the direction of stroke healing.

Pacing and proper relaxation are vital; activity and rest need to be balanced. Short relaxation breaks unfold out across the day and keeping off excessive exertion can also help manipulate fatigue levels.

Techniques for keeping power encompass adopting appropriate frame mechanics, breaking down normal responsibilities into smaller, more potential duties, and the use of assistive era.

Emotional problems:

Depression and anxiety: A stroke may additionally have a main emotional toll. Early on within the rehabilitation device, melancholy, grief, tension, and fear are not unusual feelings.

Support agencies and counseling: Attending remedy or counseling sessions may additionally additionally assist you confront and control emotional problems. Support companies offer a venue for interplay with humans who've lengthy beyond via comparable opinions, growing a enjoy of connection and records.

Medication: In some situations, docs may additionally moreover additionally advise medicine to treat depression or anxiety signs and signs and symptoms. A clinical professional need to be consulted to get maintain of an accurate assessment and guidelines.

Emotional Liability: Following a stroke, humans may additionally additionally enjoy emotional crook duty, it truly is characterized via the usage of manner of abrupt temper swings and uncontrollable sobbing or laughter. Stroke survivors and their caregivers can also discover the ones emotional outbursts scary.

Support and information: Family individuals and caregivers need to get schooling about emotional vulnerability and the manner it pertains to stroke recuperation. The stroke survivor can control those emotional shifts with persistence, information, and truth.

Relaxation techniques: Using rest techniques, which incorporates deep breathing wearing activities, meditation, or taking element in thrilling hobbies and sports activities, will allow you to manipulate your feelings.

Loss and Adjustment: The aftermath of a stroke frequently requires large adjustments in masses of areas of existence, collectively with jobs, relationships, and daily sports.

SOCIAL SUPPORT SYSTEM BUILDING

For each stroke survivor and their cherished ones, the early levels of recuperation from a stroke can be tough and daunting. A strong manual community is important for adjusting to the physical, emotional, and cognitive adjustments that accompany a stroke. Creating a assist network at some point of this vital time can offer precious beneficial beneficial aid, idea, and motivation. In this segment, we'll go through the price of constructing a assist network and provide concrete recommendation for surviving the preliminary stages of stroke recovery.

Understanding the Value of a Support Network: A manual network is a set of individuals who provide the stroke victim emotional, bodily, and realistic manual. This community can also moreover include close to cherished ones, near friends, medical professionals, and help networks. The useful resource network is critical for accelerating recuperation and enhancing the stroke survivor's preferred nicely-being. Creating a guide community is vital at some stage within the preliminary degrees of stroke recovery for the following primary reasons:

Support on an emotional diploma: Recovering from a stroke may be stressful. It may be simpler to cope with emotions of isolation, resentment, and disappointment if you have a community of pals and circle of relatives who're know-how of your situation and empathize along with your struggles as a stroke survivor. To offer emotional useful resource, you may listen, encourage, and create a everyday environment in which to perform that.

Physical help is needed at a few stage inside the early levels of stroke rehabilitation due to the fact a few humans can also have bodily limitations that make every day duties hard.

Personal care, transportation to scientific appointments, and help with mobility are all subjects that a reliable assist network can help with. Having truthful humans help with the ones obligations no longer great encourages independence however moreover lowers the opportunity of problems.

Information & Resources: Understanding the numerous aspects of stroke rehabilitation and navigating the healthcare tool may be intimidating. A beneficial aid community can offer useful expertise, resources, and direction. This may additionally furthermore entail setting the stroke survivor in contact with medical examiners, rehabilitation programs, and assist corporations that target stroke recovery.

Motivation and encouragement: Long-term remedy and nutritional changes are regularly required for stroke recovery. A stroke survivor's desire and tenacity can be substantially advanced through having a aid machine that gives idea, encouragement, and knowledge of ledges improvement. Family and friends' encouragement can hold you inspired and provide you with a feel of purpose even as you undergo your rehabilitation.

Creating a Support Network: The following are a few conceivable movements to recollect whilst developing a help network inside the early stages of stroke restoration:

Open and sincere communication with circle of relatives and friends is crucial. Discuss the stroke's results, the restoration method, and the precise assist required. Encourage your loved ones to voice their worries, ask questions, and provide their assist.

Engage Medical Staff: Develop a dating with a scientific personnel that makes a speciality of stroke healing. They can provide beneficial advice, maintain song of improvement, and endorse the exceptional therapy and rehabilitation plans. Coordination of the recuperation machine is ensured through regular reference to medical examiners.

Join Support Groups: Finding beneficial resource businesses can provide you with a enjoy of belonging and a place to alternate testimonies with people who've had similar struggles. Support organizations, whether they be on line or in man or woman, can provide emotional help, beneficial steerage, and a steady putting for speaking about issues and asking questions.

Utilize Technology: In the digital generation of nowadays, technology may be a key factor of creating a beneficial resource community. Online system, cell applications, and wearable tech can be used to expose improvement, communicate with scientific professionals, and get right of entry to instructional substances and online assist networks.

Professional Counseling: If you or a loved one has actually suffered a stroke, reflect onconsideration on getting expert counseling services, collectively with remedy or counseling. Any highbrow fitness issues, coping mechanisms, and adjustment to the changes introduced on by way of the usage of stroke healing may be facilitated with expert care.

Building a beneficial useful resource community may be surprisingly beneficial and galvanizing whilst navigating the early tiers of stroke restoration.

REHABILITATION APPROACHES FOR STROKE RECOVERY.

USE OF PHYSICAL THERAPY TO REGAIN STRENGTH AND MOBILITY

In the recuperation method for those who have had a stroke, physical therapy is important. In stroke survivors, physical treatment seeks to regain their electricity, mobility, and functional independence.

The important aim of bodily treatment for stroke rehabilitation is to growth the affected person's mobility and capacity for every day living sports. It entails an extensive assessment of the affected character's bodily competencies, constraints, and desires, which office work the cornerstone of making a personalized remedy plan.

Initial Evaluation: In step one, the bodily therapist evaluates the affected person's present beneficial abilities, which incorporates electricity, range of movement, stability, coordination, and gait. They look at any modern discomfort or sensory impairments as well.

Goal-putting: The bodily therapist establishes unique, quantifiable goals for the rehabilitation approach primarily based on the initial assessment and in session with the affected person. These targets may also additionally encompass improving coordination, fostering independence in each day life obligations, growing range of motion, restoring energy, and enhancing stability.

Exercises for mobilization and sort of motion are performed with the affected man or woman's assist with the useful resource of manner of the physical therapist to avoid muscle stiffness and joint contractures. To hold joint flexibility, those bodily sports include gently extending the form of motion within the affected limbs.

Exercises for Strengthening: Weakness is a ordinary facet impact of stroke. Specific muscle corporations injured with the resource of the stroke are the focal point of the tailor-made power schooling packages created through physical therapists. To regularly build energy and decorate all-spherical sensible skills, they employ a number of techniques which incorporates resistance bands, weights, and isometric workout workouts.

Training in Balance and Coordination: Stroke patients frequently conflict with their stability and coordination, which may additionally cause them to much more likely to fall. Exercises utilized by physical therapists are designed to test and enhance those capabilities. This can entail executing specific coordination drills, moving your weight round, and standing on choppy surfaces.

Chapter 5: Occupational Therapy For Personal Suitability

For those laid low with a stroke, occupational remedy (OT) for every day residing skills is an critical rehabilitation method. Occupational treatment's goal is to assist stroke sufferers reclaim their independence and decorate their ability to perform sports of each day residing (ADLs), together with mobility, self-care, and house responsibilities.

A character's functionality to perform each day duties can be drastically impacted through the bodily, cognitive, and sensory impairments which are regularly added on with the useful resource of stroke. By treating the ones deficits and supporting humans in regaining purposeful capacities, occupational therapists who concentrate on stroke rehabilitation play a crucial role in accelerating the restoration method.

An outline of approaches occupational treatment emphasizes every day lifestyles abilties to resource stroke recovery is provided here:

Assessment: The occupational therapist starts offevolved with the aid of the usage of acting an extensive evaluation to apprehend the individual's strengths, weaknesses, and objectives. This assessment seems at someone's motor skills, stability, coordination, sensory capabilities, cognition, and emotional fitness. The therapist can create a custom remedy plan via studying the stroke survivor's specific problems.

Self-Care Training: Self-care is one of the foremost subjects protected in occupational treatment. This covers responsibilities together with washing, clothing, grooming, feeding, and the usage of the restroom. To inspire independence in the ones sports activities activities, the therapist may additionally moreover hire an entire lot of strategies such as adaptive generation. They would in all likelihood discuss one-handed techniques, assistive gadgets like draw close bars, adaptive garments, or especially designed cutlery as approaches to make amends for bodily constraints.

Mobility Training: Hemiplegia/hemiparesis, a situation wherein one element of the body is susceptible or paralyzed after a stroke, isn't always unusual. To increase independence in on foot, transfers (together with from mattress to chair), and hiking stairs, occupational therapists recognition on enhancing stability and mobility. To encourage stable and effective strolling, they may hire recuperation physical video video games, assistive equipment (which consist of canes and walkers), and gait schooling techniques.

Cognitive Rehabilitation: Strokes can also effect someone's govt, memory, interest, and trouble-fixing capabilities. To enhance these talents, occupational therapists use cognitive rehabilitation techniques in ordinary obligations. Improve making plans and organisation skills, this may entail memorizing strategies, schooling sustained interest, and training venture sequencing.

Adaptive Approaches and Equipment: To make up for bodily or cognitive barriers, occupational therapists also can endorse the use of assistive generation or introducing adaptive techniques. For example, they might advocate tailored utensils, included handles, or reaching aids to promote beneficial independence or educate power conservation practices to lessen weariness in some unspecified time in the future of everyday sports activities activities.

Occupational therapists evaluate the stroke survivor's home environment and make hints for modifications to enhance protection and accessibility. To facilitate movement and save you falls, this could entail advising the installation of handrails, take preserve of bars, wheelchair ramps, or rearranging fixtures. People can also restore self guarantee and independence in their nonpublic homes with the useful resource of changing the surroundings.

Community Reintegration: Occupational treatment additionally places a robust emphasis on assisting stroke sufferers in finding extremely good employment and reintegrating into their companies. The abilties required for going lower back to work, interacting with others, or following pastimes and hobbies may be addressed through therapists. This may additionally need to entail learning a exchange, improving social competencies, and discovering new pastimes.

Occupational therapists art work closely with stroke survivors, their households, and a multidisciplinary employer of medical experts, which incorporates physiotherapists, psychologists, and speech therapists, in the course of the rehabilitation way. Through this teamwork, a whole approach to stroke rehabilitation is ensured, contemplating the man or woman's physical, cognitive, emotional, and social properly-being.

It's critical to keep in mind that occupational remedy interventions for stroke rehabilitation are very customized and rely upon the proper necessities and goals of every body. Progress is possible irrespective of the remedy's period or degree of intensity.

THERAPY OF SPEECH AND LANGUAGE FOR RESTORATION OF COMMUNICATION

For the ones who have had a stroke and are having communication issues, speech and language remedy (SLT) is an important a part of the rehabilitation method. A stroke is a systematic sickness that occurs while there can be an interruption inside the blood go along with the glide to the mind, causing harm to fine elements of the thoughts. Speaking, decoding, analyzing, and writing are just a few of the communique-associated issues that could cease end result from this impairment.

The main intention of speech and language remedy for stroke rehabilitation is to useful resource humans in regaining their capability for effective communique. This gadget entails an in depth assessment of the individual's communicative capabilities as well as expertise of the right stroke-affected regions. A customized therapy approach will then be created with the useful resource of the therapist to address these communication issues and sell healing.

Aphasia is one of the critical areas of emphasis in SLT for stroke recuperation. Aphasia is a language state of affairs that could boom after a stroke and impair someone's capability for verbal expression further to comprehension of spoken and written language. To supply a lift to language abilties, the speech therapist will use a number of strategies and physical video games, which encompass word retrieval sporting events, sentence manufacturing bodily video games, and studying comprehension assignments. When speech is notably broken, they'll additionally use augmentative and alternative communique (AAC) techniques, collectively with the usage of conversation forums or gadgets, to facilitate conversation.

Dysarthria is some one-of-a-kind detail of communique that a stroke may additionally effect. A motor speech trouble referred to as dysarthria is delivered on via weakened or paralyzed speech-producing muscle tissues. It may bring about slurred speech, hassle pronouncing terms, and faded vocal amount. Through strategies consisting of breath manipulate sports activities sports, tongue and lip sporting activities, and vocalization drills, the speech therapist will try to deliver a lift to the muscle mass applied in speech manufacturing and decorate articulation.

SLT for stroke rehabilitation can also additionally attention on cognitive-verbal exchange issues similarly to addressing aphasia and dysarthria. Stroke can regulate cognitive techniques like attention, memory, problem-fixing, and government functioning, which could impair verbal and written communication. To assist humans regain cognitive-communique talents, the speech therapist can also use cognitive retraining sports activities activities, memory techniques, and trouble-fixing sports activities activities.

Additionally, conversation is a social hobby, and social interaction and pragmatic language competencies are both significantly impacted with the aid of stroke. Therapy classes focusing on improving social verbal exchange skills, which incorporates flip-taking, preserving eye contact, and decoding non-verbal signs and symptoms, likely a difficulty of SLT for stroke rehabilitation. The therapist can also offer guidance and help to help humans address the emotional and mental consequences of conversation worrying conditions as a result of a stroke.

Remember that speech and language remedy for stroke recovery is a group try related to the patient, their family, and the multidisciplinary rehabilitation group. To gain an intensive and protected approach to rehabilitation, the therapist will collaborate closely with different healthcare specialists like occupational therapists, physical therapists, and neuropsychologists.

Overall, the rehabilitation gadget for those enhancing from a stroke must consist of speech and language remedy. SLT can assist humans reclaim their functionality for self-expression, know-how of others, and appealing in exciting social interactions, thereby enhancing their number one awesome of lifestyles.

MENTORING AND SUPPORT FROM PSYCHOLOGISTS

The rehabilitation system for stroke restoration is notably aided via using mental help and treatment. A stroke, regularly known as a "mind attack," also can have a excessive horrible impact on one's bodily, emotional, and intellectual fitness. Physical barriers, cognitive impairments, temper and persona modifications, adjustment problems, and other troubles can all upward push up after a stroke. At this element, counseling and intellectual help are critical elements of the rehabilitation approach.

Taking Care of Emotional Distress: Stroke survivors regularly revel in an entire lot of feelings, which encompass melancholy, fear, worry, anger, frustration, and loss. These feelings can be delivered on with the beneficial aid of the abrupt adjustments of their lives, the lack of their freedom, or the demanding situations associated with adjusting to bodily limits. Psychological assistance and therapy provide humans a steady putting in which to precise and device their emotions, supporting them in growing suitable coping mechanisms to address emotional ache.

Facilitating Adjustment and Coping: Recovery from a stroke necessitates huge modifications in an entire lot of sides of life, together with every day exercises, interpersonal interactions, and self-identification. Counseling offers direction, help, and useful coping mechanisms to help stroke survivors in navigating these transitions. It permits humans set realistic desires, decorate their functionality to treatment problems and boom their resilience in order to face any boundaries they'll face at some point of the recuperation system.

Enhancing Self-Esteem and Confidence: Stroke survivors also can experience a decline in arrogance and self notion due to bodily limits, cosmetic modifications, or worrying situations in completing duties they as soon as excelled at. Psychological help and remedy help people in figuring out their property, regaining self-assurance of their skills, and developing a notable self-picture. To assist stroke sufferers feel completed and deserving of themselves, therapists artwork with them to find out and apprehend their accomplishments.

Taking Care of Cognitive Challenges: Strokes can cause cognitive impairments like reminiscence loss, interest deficits, and issues with trouble-solving and choice-making. To cope with those issues, counseling may also use cognitive rehabilitation techniques. To fortify cognitive strategies and considerable cognitive properly-being, therapists may moreover additionally use techniques together with memory drills, hobby schooling, and hassle-fixing physical activities.

Supporting carers: Psychological help and remedy are useful for stroke survivors' carers as a whole lot as for the survivors themselves. The emotional and physical needs of being concerned for a stroke survivor can bring about caregiver strain, fatigue, and intellectual health troubles. Counseling offers carers a stable place to voice their concerns, find out suitable coping mechanisms, and get advice at the manner to address the troubles of caregiving.

Promoting Lifestyle Changes: Making huge manner of life changes, which include switching to a more in form food regimen, exercising regularly, and getting to know to control pressure, are regularly crucial for stroke restoration. When it includes inspiring and assisting humans in engaging in those changes, intellectual manual and counseling can be extremely beneficial. Therapists can help stroke survivors and their families installation and hold healthful residing conduct with the aid of using offering understanding, equipment, and persevering with useful resource.

Building Social Support: Stroke survivors may enjoy social isolation and loneliness because of the reality they'll locate it hard to socialize because of bodily or conversation barriers. Psychological assist and counseling can assist people in re-installing place their social networks, enhancing their verbal exchange abilties, and creating plans for having fruitful social interactions. To promote a enjoy of community and peer help, therapists might also moreover lead resource corporations or connect stroke survivors with close by assets.

Counseling and intellectual help are important factors of the rehabilitation method for stroke recovery. They interest at the social, emotional, and mental components of stroke survivors' lives, assisting them in overcoming barriers introduced on with the aid of the usage of their disorder, mastering coping mechanisms, regaining self warranty, and improving their fashionable properly-being. The recovery and great of existence of stroke survivors are extensively aided through the use of psychological help and counseling because they provide an in depth and all-encompassing method to rehabilitation after a stroke.

ADDRESSING COGNITIVE AND EMOTIONAL CHANGES IS COVERED

REHABILITATION OF THE MINDFUL AND IMPROVEMENT OF MEMORY

The aim of cognitive rehabilitation and reminiscence improvement is to aid human beings in regaining cognitive function and improving their reminiscence after a stroke. Strokes can purpose numerous cognitive troubles, which incorporates reminiscence loss, attention deficiencies, hassle making selections, and reminiscence loss. Strokes arise at the same time as the blood supply to the mind is cut off. Programs for cognitive rehabilitation are created to deal with the ones deficiencies and encourage the recovery of cognitive capability.

Understanding Cognitive Rehabilitation: The aim of cognitive rehabilitation is to retrain and restore cognitive talents which have been damaged with the useful resource of a stroke. It includes some of strategies, drills, and sports catered to the proper requirements of absolutely everyone. Enhancing cognitive capacities, growing useful independence, and facilitating reintegration into regular lifestyles are the goals.

Techniques for Improving Memory: Memory issues are from time to time a prevent end result of a stroke. Techniques for memory improvement are used to assist people become better at encoding, storing, and retrieving statistics. These techniques embody:

a. External memory aids: These equipment provide outdoor assistance to make up for reminiscence deficits. Calendars, reminder apps, notebooks, and digital gadgets with records storage and retrieval abilities are some examples.

b. Internal reminiscence strategies: These strategies educate people at the way to enhance their reminiscence. Mnemonic strategies collectively with chunking, association, and visualization can help with reminiscence encoding and retrieval.

Chapter 6: Emotional Assimilations And Coping Methods

Recovery from a stroke is a difficult and complex system that calls for no longer sincerely bodily remedy but moreover coping mechanisms and emotional variations. Since strokes may additionally want to have a extremely good impact on a person's highbrow fitness and emotional scenario, emotional nicely-being is vital to the general rehabilitation process. Understanding and handling the ones emotional changes are essential for encouraging complete healing and raising the same antique of dwelling for stroke survivors.

Following a stroke, human beings regularly warfare with an entire lot of emotional problems, which include disappointment, despair, worry, frustration, anger, and a feel of loss. These feelings may be a surrender stop result of severa topics, which incorporates the suddenness and unpredictability of the stroke, any bodily limits that might take a look at, the worry about future strokes, and the subsequent modifications in life-style and diploma of independence.

Stroke survivors can use a lot of techniques to deal with those emotional changes:

Finding emotional help: Talking to friends, cherished ones, guide groups, or therapists who are familiar with the problems of stroke rehabilitation may be a amazing way to find out emotional aid. Sharing mind and feelings with others who have lengthy lengthy past via similar tales may also need to make stroke survivors experience heaps much less by myself and further understood.

Acceptance and adjustment: A essential section in emotional recovery is coming to grips with the effects of the stroke and accepting the modifications it has added about. This involves accepting constraints and adjusting to novel conditions. A greater resilient mind-set may be attained with the resource of the use of adopting a effective mindset and that specialize in what remains feasible in preference to lamenting past disasters.

Therapy: Attending man or woman or commercial enterprise company remedy schooling, which incorporates counseling or cognitive-behavioral therapy, can assist stroke sufferers deal with their feelings. Therapists can assist sufferers in recognizing terrible notion styles, acquiring coping mechanisms, and processing loss and grief. Additionally, remedy sessions provide a strong putting for expressing emotions and growing green coping mechanisms.

Physical interest and rehabilitation: Taking element in the ones sports and applications no longer amazing helps the frame heal bodily, however it additionally has a awesome effect on the mind and spirit. Exercise regularly releases endorphins, which can be organic temper enhancers. Achieving bodily rehabilitation milestones can also increase self warranty and preferred shallowness.

Maintaining a healthy way of life: Emotional adjustment and coping mechanisms require which you preserve a notable diet, get enough sleep, and manipulate your strain tiers. The body's herbal recuperation strategies are supported via a healthy healthy dietweight-reduction plan and enough sleep, and pressure-good deal techniques like mindfulness, meditation, and rest bodily games can help lower anxiety and decorate emotional nicely-being.

Realistic intention-placing is crucial for stroke survivors, as is concentrated on small victories. Larger dreams may be damaged down into greater potential, ability steps to reduce feelings of crush and decorate motivation. A revel in of success and optimism can be generated through acknowledging every accomplishment alongside the direction.

Getting used to new conditions: Recovery from a stroke regularly consists of getting used to new each day sporting activities, abilities, and duties. Stroke patients can advantage freedom and enhance their emotional well-being with the aid of the usage of seeking out assist gadgets, changing their dwelling state of affairs, or gaining statistics of latest skills.

It's crucial to do not forget that each stroke survivor's stories and desires are without a doubt one in all a type, for that reason emotional adjustment and coping mechanisms can also moreover variety from character to man or woman. After a stroke, a entire technique that consists of counseling, emotional guide, bodily restoration, and proper way of lifestyles choices can lay a sturdy basis for emotional recovery.

MANAGING POST-STROKE ANXIETY AND DEPRESSION

Anxiety and publish-stroke disappointment are commonplace mental problems which could have an effect on humans who have had a stroke. A stroke, a medical emergency that occurs whilst blood float to the mind is interrupted, may have extraordinary horrible physical, emotional, and intellectual affects. According to estimates, approximately one-zero.33 of stroke survivors display signs and symptoms of depression, and a comparable variety also can display symptoms of anxiety.

Understanding Post-Stroke Sadness and Anxiety: Although they may be separate issues, publish-stroke disappointment, and tension often coexist and may have a extraordinary poor have an impact on on a stroke survivor's sizeable nicely-being and exceptional of existence. The bodily and intellectual effects of the stroke itself, changes in thoughts chemistry, and troubles adjusting to existence after a stroke are just a few reasons of these ailments.

Post-stroke depression stocks many symptoms with medical melancholy, which includes persistent unhappiness, hopelessness, lack of hobby in as soon as-interesting sports, modifications in appetite and sleep patterns, exhaustion, problem concentrating, and suicidal or self-harming mind. Additionally, bodily symptoms and symptoms like unexplained ache, intestinal troubles, or complications may also moreover seem in stroke survivors who furthermore have melancholy.

Post-stroke anxiety signs and symptoms and symptoms embody immoderate worry, restlessness, irritability, trouble unwinding, and problem snoozing, as well as physical manifestations which incorporates fast heartbeat, shortness of breath, or trembling. Additionally, it can result in progressed anxiety or dread of having each other stroke or of experiencing limits in regular sports.

Managing Depression and Anxiety after a Stroke:

Medical examination: It is important to looking for a scientific exam from healthcare professionals, collectively with neurologists, psychiatrists, or psychologists if a stroke survivor famous signs and symptoms of despair or anxiety. They can determine the condition's severity and create a appropriate remedy technique.

Medication: To deal with symptoms, scientific doctors may additionally supply antidepressants or anxiety drugs. Inhibitors of selective serotonin reuptake (SSRIs) are frequently given for put up-stroke melancholy because of their performance and commonly favorable detail outcomes. Remedy is often paired with additional treatment plans due to the fact it may not be sufficient to take treatment by myself.

Psychotherapy: Using cognitive-behavioral remedy (CBT), a form of talk remedy, may be very useful in treating post-stroke disappointment and anxiety. CBT assists human beings in recognizing and converting unhelpful idea patterns, acquiring coping mechanisms, and addressing emotional and behavioral problems. Additionally, psychotherapy offers stroke survivors a constant region to vent their feelings and troubles, fostering mental recovery and resilience.

Supportive Interventions: A fashion of supportive interventions may be used alongside aspect remedy and drugs. These must encompass guide businesses wherein stroke survivors can meet human beings going thru similar issues and exchange stories. Furthermore, occupational remedy, physical remedy, and speech remedy can boost up recuperation after a stroke, growth self notion, and lessen depressive or annoying signs and signs and symptoms and signs and signs.

Lifestyle Modifications: Healthy way of life modifications can help lessen post-stroke despair and anxiety. A wholesome manner of lifestyles includes everyday exercise, a nicely-balanced eating regimen, sufficient sleep, and abstinence from drugs and alcohol. Maintaining a social existence and taking element in a laugh sports activities can also help to enhance highbrow fitness and reduce feelings of loneliness.

Support from caregivers: To assist stroke survivors who are depressed and irritating, caregivers are extremely essential. They need to be knowledgeable approximately the situations, covered in the remedy desire way, and given machine for stress manipulate. The intellectual and physical duties of caregiving may be managed via caregivers with the useful resource of aid businesses or counseling.

Continuity of Care: Treating tension and sadness following a stroke takes time. Follow-up visits with scientific specialists are required to tune development, regulate tablets as appropriate, and offer non-save you manual and direction.

SEEKING ASSISTANCE FROM PROFESSIONALS IN MENTAL HEALTH

During the healing from a stroke, in search of assist from intellectual fitness professionals may be pretty useful in supporting human beings in managing those emotional problems and facilitating their sizable recovery and rehabilitation. Psychologists, schizophrenics, and precise intellectual health professionals can offer specialized direction, assist, and healing interventions to fulfill the precise requirements of stroke survivors.

The following are some essential regions in which highbrow fitness practitioners can beneficial aid stroke survivors:

Emotional stability: Mental fitness professionals can resource stroke sufferers in navigating the emotional united statesand downs that frequently accompany the restoration manner. They deliver people an area in which they are able to unique all in their feelings, collectively with sadness, rage, and different terrible feelings. They can assist human beings in developing coping mechanisms, hard unfavorable notion patterns, and fostering emotional resilience thru lots of restoration techniques, which encompass cognitive-behavioral remedy (CBT) or reputation and determination treatment (ACT).

Adjustment and coping strategies: After a stroke, it may be tough to regulate to the bodily and way of lifestyles changes. When developing green coping mechanisms which can be precise to genuinely all and sundry's situation, intellectual fitness specialists can offer help. They can offer advice on a way to cope with every day sports activities sports, alter to bodily regulations, and growth a modern day experience of self and purpose.

Motivation for rehabilitation: Recovery after a stroke frequently entails top notch art work and tenacity. For their rehabilitation adventure, people can get inspired and set manageable dreams with the useful resource of intellectual fitness experts. To make sure a holistic method to restoration, they might provide guide, assist in identifying strengths, and collaborate with other healthcare experts.

Support and education for the circle of relatives are vital because of the truth getting better from a stroke influences not top notch the affected individual but moreover their carers and circle of relatives. By guiding them thru the emotional outcomes of the stroke, coaching them at the rehabilitation system, and fostering conversation and coping mechanisms in the own family unit, highbrow health specialists can help circle of relatives members.

Chapter 7: Adaptive Equipment And Mobility Assistants

By providing humans guide, balance, and assist as they are trying to regain their independence, mobility aids, and adaptive devices play a essential function in accelerating stroke restoration. These equipment are supposed to assist stroke survivors enhance their mobility, balance, and capability to carry out daily sports (ADLs), in order to decorate their common brilliant of lifestyles.

Walking Aids: Stroke patients regularly make use of on foot aids to regain their ability to stroll securely and effectively. Among those gear are:

Canes: Canes provide stability and manual to humans who have slight stability issues. When one facet of the frame is weaker than the opportunity, it may be specifically beneficial.

Walkers: Compared to canes, walkers provide more stability and useful resource. They are useful for people who need more aid with their stability and weight-bearing. Standard walkers, wheeled walkers, and rollators are some of the numerous sorts of walkers.

Crutches: People who need to preserve weight off one or each of their legs use crutches. They beneficial beneficial useful resource in equilibrium in the direction of the healing technique and provide resource.

Wheelchairs: For stroke patients who've big mobility regulations or are not able to walk, wheelchairs are crucial mobility aids. They offer people freedom and give the opportunity for them to transport round quite simply. Depending on the man or woman's unique desires and talents, wheelchairs might be powered or guide. Additionally, they'll encompass diverse customization talents like adjustable chairs and particular cushions to increase consolation and avoid stress sores.

Orthotic gadgets are used to useful useful resource paralyzed or prone limbs, increase mobility, and keep away from joint contractures. Examples of these devices embody braces and splints. To offer most suitable alignment and assist, those devices are in my view ready. To help with practical motion and save you muscular stiffness, orthotic devices may be used on the lower extremities (ankle-foot orthoses) or the pinnacle extremities (hand and wrist splints).

Transfer Aids: Moving from a mattress to a wheelchair or from a wheelchair to a automobile may be tough for stroke survivors. Transfer aids make the ones moves easier and assist preserve protection. Transfer boards, sliding sheets, switch belts, and mechanical lifts are a few examples of switch aids. These gadgets now not handiest assist in transfers however additionally lessen the danger of falls and accidents at the same time as doing so.

Activities of Daily Living (ADLs) Adaptive Devices: Stroke sufferers also can revel in problems with some of ADLs, which include dressing, bathing, eating, and grooming. These problems are addressed and independence is recommended with the aid of using adaptive generation. Several instances include:

Dressing aids: These assist with manipulating clothing fasteners and consist of elastic shoelaces, button hooks, and zipper pulls.

Bathing aids: Grab bars, bathe seats, and prolonged-treated sponges make it extra consistent for people to wash and hold themselves smooth.

Eating aids: For stroke patients with hand weakness or constrained dexterity, adaptive utensils with big handles, angled or weighted utensils, and plate protectors make it much less hard for them to feed themselves.

Grooming aids: Tools like electric powered toothbrushes, extended-treated combs, and adaptable nail clippers help stroke sufferers keep their grooming and cleanliness.

It is vital to keep in thoughts that deciding on mobility assistance or a chunk of tailor-made tool should be based definitely mostly on the needs and abilties of the character. Each stroke survivor's specific goals may be evaluated by using the usage of way of a healthcare expert, which includes a bodily therapist or occupational therapist, who can then endorse the first rate enables to assist them on their street to recovery. As the character advances of their rehabilitation and as their desires modify over time, habitual re-evaluation and machine adjustment can also be required.

AAC DEVICES: AUGMENTATIVE AND ALTERNATIVE COMMUNICATION

AAC (Augmentative and Alternative Communication) gadget help humans speak while speech or language is impaired due to a stroke or unique clinical state of affairs. By giving people a manner to express themselves, improve their conversation talents, and enhance their contemporary remarkable of lifestyles, those gadgets play a massive issue in stroke recuperation. We shall dig into the specifics of AAC gadgets for stroke healing in this reaction.

Understanding Stroke and Communication Impairment: A stroke takes region at the same time as there may be a disruption within the blood flow to the thoughts, which motives harm to precise elements of the brain. Individuals might also revel in a whole lot of conversation problems depending on the kind and place of the stroke. A commonplace language problem called aphasia diminishes someone's potential for records and speakme. Additionally, a motor making plans hassle called apraxia of speech, which disrupts the coordination of speakme actions, can get up. Another viable outcome is dysarthria, wherein the muscles accountable for generating speech are tormented by muscle weak point or paralysis.

AAC devices are purported to useful aid or take the place of spoken verbal exchange for people who've problem expressing themselves verbally. These machine are intended to promote independence, enhance communique, and reduce frustration. They offer particular methods to specific ideas, desires, and feelings. AAC system can be quite useful for regaining and improving verbal exchange capabilities in stroke patients.

AAC Device Types:

a. Picture-Based Systems: In the ones structures, terms, sentences, and mind are represented by way of the usage of using pix or symbols. To deliver their message, human beings can also either select the proper pictures or issue at them. Communication packages, message boards, and photograph alternate conversation structures (PECS) are some examples.

b. SGDs, or speech-producing devices, are digital equipment that produce speech primarily based mostly on man or woman enter. They can variety from handheld gadgets to pill-based totally sincerely packages, and that they may be configured with several vocabulary opportunities. To talk, users can select pictures, enter messages, or utilize pre-programmed terms.

c. Software that turns typed or written text into speech is known as text-to-speech. Stroke survivors can speak with the useful aid of typing messages on computer systems, tablets, or smartphones with this period.

d. Eye-Gaze Systems: These current-day AAC gadget display screen the man or woman's eye movement to check the alternatives they need to make. Users can speak thru focusing their eyes on the famous alternative even as navigating through a grid of symbols or phrases.

AAC Devices' Stroke Recovery Benefits

a. Improved Communication: AAC device deliver stroke sufferers a manner to speak truly, promoting communique and social connection.

b. Language Rehabilitation: The use of AAC machine as a remedy tool can help humans regain their language capabilities. The tool lets in stroke sufferers to exercise phrase retrieval, sentence manufacturing, and different language capabilities.

c. Greater Independence: By minimizing a person's dependency on specific people for communication, AAC gadgets empower customers. They can reclaim their every day enjoy of autonomy and control.

d. Support for Caregivers: By selling superior communication and minimizing misconceptions, AAC gadgets help reduce the burden on caregivers. Improved care can quit result from caregivers having a more expertise of the goals and picks of stroke survivors.

AAC devices can be custom designed to in shape the proper necessities and competencies of stroke survivors. They may be custom designed with particular vocabulary, expressions which can be regularly used, and desired verbal exchange techniques. To make use of AAC devices efficaciously, training and assist also are critical. AAC experts and speech-language pathologists can provide recommendation on device desire, customization, and schooling techniques.

For stroke sufferers with communique issues, augmentative and opportunity communique era are useful property. These equipment facilitate stroke recuperation, improve conversation, promote independence, and beautify notable of life average via presenting numerous modes of expression. AAC gadgets preserve to increase with everyday technological breakthroughs, presenting increasingly more inexperienced options for human beings on their path.

ADVANCES IN TECHNOLOGY FOR COGNITIVE REHABILITATION

With contemporary and robust approaches to beautify cognitive function and top notch of existence for stroke survivors, technological improvements in cognitive rehabilitation have had a large impact on stroke healing. Memory loss, recognition troubles, language issues, and government characteristic issues are just a few of the cognitive impairments that can quit result from stroke, a neurological contamination added on with the aid of blood go with the float troubles in the mind. Traditional cognitive rehabilitation techniques require monotonous carrying events and treatment classes, however technological upgrades have completely changed this case via introducing interactive and individualized procedures.

Virtual Reality (VR): VR technology has end up a high-quality beneficial useful resource inside the remedy of stroke. VR technology creates interactive, realistic environments that mimic real-global conditions in order that stroke sufferers can participate in rehabilitation sports. VR can be used to beautify quite some cognitive techniques, inclusive of govt feature, hobby, and reminiscence. For instance, interactive video video games and simulations in virtual reality environments may be created to test game enthusiasts' recollection, recognition, and desire-making abilities.

Serious Games: Also referred to as gamified rehabilitation, severe video video games harness the capability of online gaming to decorate cognitive rehabilitation. The cognitive troubles that stroke sufferers frequently stumble upon are the point of interest of those video video games. Serious video video games offer a amusing platform for healing wearing sports activities that encourages sufferers to exercising cognitive capabilities engagingly. Specific cognitive abilities like hobby, reminiscence, problem-solving, and language may be centered by way of using the video games.

Brain-Computer Interfaces (BCIs): Cognitive rehabilitation for stroke healing has demonstrated considerable promise even as the usage of brain-computer interfaces. BCIs create an immediate line of communication between the mind and extracellular devices, allowing stroke sufferers to feature virtual interfaces with their brainwaves. This generation may be used for numerous activities, together with managing virtual worlds, gambling video video games, or perhaps facilitating conversation. BCIs also can be achieved to offer real-time remarks on thoughts interest, supporting patients and clinical specialists in tracking the improvement and enhancing remedy plans as important.

Wearable Technology: In cognitive rehabilitation, wearable generation—which includes smartwatches and health trackers—has acquired recognition. Heart charge, sleep styles, and tiers of physical interest are just a few of the physiological statistics that those gadgets can track and keep a watch on. Healthcare vendors can studies greater approximately a affected individual's favored well-being and cognitive fitness by means of way of the use of collecting statistics on those parameters. Wearable era can also characteristic a reminder or prompt for taking medicinal capsules, attending appointments, and acting physical treatment carrying sports, supporting stroke patients on their road to recuperation.

Technologies that allow humans with disabilities in their each day sports activities are called assistive technologies. Smart domestic structures, voice-activated assistants, prescription manipulate apps, and digital conversation aids are some of those technology. Stroke sufferers who use the ones generation during their healing can restore their independence and sharpen their cognitive competencies.

Remote rehabilitation has turn out to be extra on hand and to be had for stroke sufferers thanks to the development of telecommunications generation. Through net structures and video chats, telemedicine permits patients to acquire a ways flung cognitive rehabilitation therapy. With this method, geographical guidelines are eliminated and those can get maintain of expert remedy at the same time as enjoyable of their very own homes. In addition to growing consolation, far off rehabilitation lowers healthcare fees and could growth affected person compliance.

Cognitive rehabilitation for stroke recuperation has lengthy beyond through a revolution manner to technological enhancements. There are absolutely more options than ever for individualized and exciting cognitive rehabilitation interventions due to virtual reality, excessive video video games, thoughts-pc interfaces, wearable technology, assistive era, and telemedicine. These inclinations deliver stroke sufferers the danger to regain cognitive characteristic, boom their super of life, and accelerate their rehabilitation in general.

Chapter 8: Technology That Is Accessible For Independent Living

By encouraging independence, permitting mobility, and facilitating conversation, available era performs a essential function in improving the high-quality of existence for stroke survivors. This section investigates severa to be had generation alternatives that useful resource stroke healing through impartial residing.

Movement Assistance: Impaired motion is one of the important problems that stroke survivors want to cope with. Innovative strategies for growing mobility and regaining independence is provided with the useful resource of handy era:

a. Mobility Aids: For individuals who war with stability and coordination, on foot frames, canes, and walkers with ergonomic designs and stability trends can be of assist. These device provide stroke sufferers more self perception at the equal time as navigating their surroundings.

b. Assisted Mobility: For stroke survivors with massive bodily impairments, powered wheelchairs, and mobility scooters are essential for improving mobility. Modern models permit unbiased movement every indoors and exterior with abilties like movable seating, joystick controls, and impediment reputation.

c. Robotic rehabilitation gadgets: Exoskeletons and robot arms help stroke sufferers regain motor manipulate and educate their injured limbs. These device deliver repetitive and targeted treatment, encouraging neuroplasticity and dashing up the healing approach.

Communication and assistive generation: Strokes can have an impact on a person's capacity to talk, making it hard for them to very well precise themselves. There are numerous methods that handy era can help communication and simplicity everyday interactions:

a. AAC (Augmentative and Alternative Communication) Devices: These equipment help stroke survivors who have hassle talking to carry their desires, mind, and emotions. They can be as primary as photo-based communique boards or as sophisticated as speech-producing generation. Text-to-speech technology, touchscreen consumer interfaces, and pre-programmed terms are all utilized by AAC gadgets to beautify verbal exchange.

b. Smart Home Technology: Virtual assistants (like the Amazon Echo or Google Home) that can be configured to carry out a whole lot of competencies, which includes regulating lights, temperature, and amusement systems, are examples of voice-controlled clever home devices. These gadgets permit stroke sufferers to utilize voice instructions to govern their surroundings, make telephone calls, and get right of entry to records, reducing their want for guide help.

c. Adaptive Keyboards and Switches: People who've had strokes and characteristic motor disabilities must discover it difficult to use regular keyboards or touchscreens. Alternatives for textual content access and laptop navigation are furnished via adaptive keyboards with larger keys, haptic remarks, and adjustable layouts, in addition to switches that can be brought on with little effort.

Support for Cognitive Functions: Strokes could have an effect on reminiscence, hobby, and hassle-solving abilities. Accessible era offers approaches to inspire independence and enhance cognitive function:

a. Apps for reminders and organisation: Mobile applications made specially for stroke sufferers will will will let you preserve song of your appointments, medicine schedules, and regular schedules. These apps offer visual cues, mission lists, and reminders to assist with organizing and go through in thoughts.

b. Interactive software application packages are available to assist with cognitive rehabilitation. These physical sports activities awareness on reminiscence, interest, problem-fixing, and language abilties. With the help of those applications, stroke survivors can accumulate specialized cognitive remedy at domestic based totally on their needs and improvement.

c. Digital voice recorders, smartphone apps, and wearable gadgets with reminder functions are all examples of virtual memory aids that might assist make up for memory loss. With the assist of those tool, stroke sufferers can reduce their need for outdoor assist by way of using keeping tune of essential facts, scheduling reminders, and getting cues to complete chores.

Accessible generation is vital for encouraging unbiased residing and raising the standard of living for stroke patients. The shape of generation available gives individualized answers for particular goals, from mobility useful resource to communique gear and cognitive useful resource tools. Accessible era's persevered improvement has the capability to enhance stroke rehabilitation even extra and allow humans to reclaim their independence in each day lifestyles.

MODIFICATIONS TO YOUR LIFESTYLE FOR LONG-TERM RECOVERY.

NUTRITION AND A HEALTHY DIET ARE CRUCIAL

It isn't possible to overestimate the rate of nutrients and an amazing healthy eating plan for convalescing after a stroke. A stroke reasons important bodily adjustments in someone, and the rehabilitation manner is significantly aided through manner of ingesting a healthy weight loss program. A balanced weight loss program enables the frame's herbal healing methods, reduces hazard elements, regulates risk elements, and fosters great health and nicely-being.

Supply of Nutrients: A stroke can damage the mind and special organs, ensuing in a whole lot of disabilities. The frame acquires the crucial building blocks for restore and recuperation even as it consumes a nutritious eating regimen high in key nutrients. Vitamins (together with weight-reduction plan C and nutrients E), minerals (together with calcium and magnesium), and omega-three fatty acids are vitamins that assist healthy thoughts characteristic with the resource of supporting in tissue restore and lowering infection.

Promotes Physical Recovery: After a stroke, right nutrients is important for promoting physical healing. It aids in restoring out of area characteristic, enhancing mobility, and regenerating muscle energy. Consuming enough protein is essential because it promotes muscle increase and repair. The eating regimen want to embody lean resources of protein together with poultry, fish, lentils, and dairy merchandise. Furthermore, some of end result, veggies, and complete grains encompass phytochemicals, antioxidants, and fiber that beneficial beneficial aid in restoration and decrease the danger of problems.

Manages Risk Factors: High blood stress, immoderate ldl ldl cholesterol, diabetes, and weight problems are a number of the hazard factors which may be frequently associated with stroke. These danger factors can be managed with a balanced diet plan, which moreover lowers the risk of having some other stroke. Blood strain and cholesterol levels may be regulated with a food plan reduced in sodium, saturated fats, trans fat, and ldl ldl cholesterol. Consuming food excessive in fiber and complex carbs will assist you manage your weight, keep sturdy blood sugar levels, and decrease your hazard of having diabetes.

Supports Mental Health: Recovery from a stroke includes each bodily and intellectual fitness. The renovation of brain health and cognitive feature is notably aided with the aid of using specific consuming. Walnuts, flaxseeds, and fatty fish all contain omega-3 fatty acids that enhance mind health and decrease the threat of cognitive decline. Berries, leafy veggies, and nuts are meals excessive in antioxidants that could guard the mind from oxidative stress and decorate highbrow usual performance.

Prevents Secondary outcomes: Following a stroke, people can be more at risk of secondary consequences such as infections, malnutrition, and swallowing problems. The hazard of illnesses is reduced and the immune device is strengthened with proper vitamins. To avoid malnutrition and assist the frame's restoration techniques, enough calorie and nutrient intake is critical. To assure stable and enough vitamins in conditions in which swallowing problems exist, a speech therapist or nutritionist also can recommend reduced textures or special diets.

Overall Health and Quality of Life: During the restoration after a stroke, preferred fitness and exceptional of life are notably impacted thru using an notable food regimen and nutrients. It aids in boosting strength degrees, reducing weariness, and improving the body's capability for restoration. A wholesome body is better able to address the highbrow and physical desires of restoration, which leads to an uplifted mood, greater motivation, and a experience of well-being.

Nutritional adequacy and a healthy diet plan are essential for stroke healing. It aids in bodily healing, controls threat elements, fosters mind fitness, averts issues, and improves popular nicely-being. A certified dietician, for instance, can provide individualized recommendation and recommendations primarily based totally mostly on a person's unique requirements, health state of affairs, and nutritional regulations.

Guidelines for bodily interest and Exercise

The recuperation and rehabilitation after a stroke rely considerably on exercise and bodily interest. They help those who've had a stroke in enhancing their energy, flexibility, coordination, cardiovascular fitness, and widespread satisfactory of existence. Exercise hints for stroke rehabilitation are created to be stable, inexperienced, and custom designed to the person's particular requirements and skills. Following a stroke, the following are a few specific suggestions for workout and bodily hobby:

Consultation with medical professionals: It is vital to are looking for recommendation from clinical medical doctors, physiotherapists, and rehabilitation professionals earlier than beginning any exercise software. They will have a observe your obstacles, look at your condition, and provide tailor-made advice depending to your unique situation.

Exercises for pretty a number movement and early mobilization: In the early degrees of stroke rehabilitation, the focal point is often positioned on the ones types of bodily sports. To prevent stiffness, beautify move, and keep flexibility, these wearing occasions address transferring the affected limbs and joints. They may additionally want to contain passive physical games even as the therapist lets in the affected man or woman pass their limbs, or energetic-assisted sports activities, wherein the patient starts shifting with some help.

Strength schooling: As the recovery after a stroke advances, this interest becomes essential. It allows each day activities, improves traditional bodily ordinary typical performance, and aids in the healing of muscular energy and characteristic. Stroke-affected muscle regions are focused with resistance education the use of weights, resistance bands, or body weight. To keep away from harm, the sports activities activities need to be completed in accurate shape and beneath the supervision of a medical practitioner.

Exercises for stability and coordination: Balance and coordination are frequently affected by stroke, which will increase the chance of falling. Exercises for balance and coordination are meant to growth stability and decrease the danger of similarly falls. These carrying activities have to entail on foot on uneven ground, standing on one leg, or project superb balance-centered sports like yoga or tai chi. Based on every person's competencies and development, a licensed therapist can lead and adjust those sports activities activities.

Exercise that increases cardiovascular fitness, staying energy, and stylish health is called cardiovascular exercise or cardio workout. Exercises like taking walks, cycling, swimming, or the usage of cardio devices raise the coronary coronary heart charge and breathing fees. Cardiovascular workout must be adjusted to the character's abilities and frequently intensified in duration and depth over time.

Exercises that exercise to each day life, at the aspect of having out of a chair, walking, or ascending stairs, are the focal point of sensible education. These exercising routines are purported to boom one's independence, sensible capacities, and capability for every day living responsibilities. Functional training, which might in all likelihood consist of education particular moves or replicating real-existence obligations, may be protected into rehabilitation intervals.

Exercises for flexibility and stretching: Stretching wearing activities assist maintain or enhance joint range of motion, prevent muscle tightness, and promote flexibility. To growth mobility and decrease the danger of contractures, they want to be completed regularly. Stretching need to be finished slowly and painlessly and can aim particular muscle corporations. An expert inside the area of drugs can suggest you at the right stretches and physical sports.

Chapter 9: Sleep And Renewal Activities

By fostering recuperation, assisting cognitive rehabilitation, and enhancing favored nicely-being, sleep and restorative activities are crucial to stroke restoration. The recovery technique is optimized and the mind's capability to get better and rewire itself is advanced through getting enough sleep and attractive in restorative sports.

Sleep is essential for stroke survivors as it permits the thoughts to consolidate recollections, repair broken tissues, and regenerate. The mind plays severa restorative tactics whilst we sleep, which include the elimination of waste materials and the consolidation of newly obtained information. The following are some vital factors approximately sleep and stroke recuperation:

a. Sleep encourages neural regeneration mechanisms, which useful resource within the rehabilitation of stroke-damaged thoughts tissue. It aids in the recuperation of lost function via the use of permitting the regeneration of neurons and the remodeling of thoughts connections.

b. Memory Consolidation: Sleep is essential for gaining knowledge of and memory development. For stroke patients present technique rehabilitation, it improves the mind's ability to method and keep new facts.

c. Stroke patients often warfare with emotional difficulties like despair and tension. Getting enough sleep can help the control of those mental troubles with the aid of the usage of using regulating temper and emotional reactions.

d. Energy Restoration: Recovery from a stroke wishes a number of bodily and emotional power. Getting sufficient sleep facilitates restore power ranges, allowing humans to participate in rehabilitation sports greater effectively.

Optimizing sleep hygiene strategies is crucial for stroke survivors to enhance the quantity and tremendous of their shut eye. Here are a few guidelines:

a. Establish a constant sleep time table by way of the use of going to mattress and waking up at the same time each day. Better sleep is endorsed and the frame's inner clock is regulated as a end result.

b. Make Your Sleep Environment Restful: Make sure your mattress room is peaceful, cushty, and distraction-unfastened. If required, use white noise generators, masks over your eyes, or earplugs.

c. Manage Light Exposure: To manage the circadian rhythm, reveal oneself to herbal mild during the day. To inspire the technology of melatonin and put together the frame for sleep inside the nighttime, dim the lighting and restriction exposure to digital gadgets that emit blue slight.

d. Regular Physical Activity: Exercise often within the direction of the day to improve your extraordinary of sleep at night time.

Consult medical examiners to understand the pleasant physical games for improving from a stroke.

e. Limit or keep away from stimulants like caffeine, nicotine, and alcohol, specially right earlier than night, as they're capable of impair the super of your sleep.

f. Practice relaxation techniques before bed to encourage a quiet and serene circumstance appropriate to sleep, together with deep respiratory physical video games, meditation, or modern muscle relaxation.

Restorative Practices for Stroke Recovery: Besides getting sufficient sleep, adopting restorative practices into your every day habitual might probably help you recover from a stroke. These strategies are intended to ease tension, encourage rest, and beautify famous well-being. Here are some instances:

a. Mindfulness and meditation: Using mindfulness and meditation strategies permit you to reduce stress, awareness more honestly, and experience higher emotionally. By decreasing the signs and symptoms and signs and symptoms of unhappiness and tension, mindfulness-based absolutely stress cut price packages have tested promise within the healing from stroke.

b. Yoga and Tai Chi: Gentle physical video games that concentrate on relaxation and stress discount, along facet yoga and tai chi, can help with stability, coordination, and flexibility. These tactics may be changed to meet the great necessities and abilities of stroke survivors.

c. Massage: Massages can relieve annoying muscle agencies, increase motion, and inspire rest. Additionally, it might be outstanding for mood and fashionable well-being.

Techniques for Managing Stress and Relaxation

The use of relaxation strategies and pressure reduce fee strategies is crucial for stroke rehabilitation. As they regulate to the physical, cognitive, and emotional modifications that accompany a stroke, stroke survivors frequently face diverse degrees of pressure, worry, and emotional issues. These dangerous emotions can be decreased, elegant properly-being can be improved, and the recovery approach may be extended through incorporating stress manipulate and rest practices into their rehabilitation plan.

Here are a few effective pressure discount and relaxation techniques that could beneficial resource in stroke recovery:

Deep breathing techniques: Deep respiratory strategies beneficial aid in relaxation and pressure cut price. Encourage stroke patients to discover a snug posture to sit down or lie down in and to take some calm, deep breaths, inhaling thru the nostril and expelling through the mouth. This approach can be used severa instances consistent with day to lower blood stress, soothe the annoying machine, and improve the oxygenation of the whole frame.

Progressive Muscle Relaxation: Using this approach, every muscle employer inside the body is sequentially tensed and then launched, starting on the feet and operating as a good deal because the pinnacle. Stroke survivors can deepen their relaxation and boom their recognition of their body's sensations via deliberately tensing and then enjoyable their muscle tissues. Progressive muscular rest can ease tension within the muscle tissues, encourage sleep, and reduce anxiety.

Guided imagery is a relaxation method that employs visualization to conjure up great highbrow snap shots to help you unwind and experience proper. Stroke sufferers might possibly art work with a therapist who leads them thru a rest script or listen to guided imagery recordings. People can reduce stress and tension and allow their our our our bodies and minds unwind via that specialize in serene and calming imagery like a serene lawn or a non violent seashore.

Focusing on the present 2nd even as accepting and acknowledging any mind, emotions, or physical sensations that come with out judgment is the motive of mindfulness meditation. Stroke survivors who discover a non violent place, take a seat or lie down in a snug function, and focus their attention on their breath or a particular sensation of their frame should in all likelihood exercise mindfulness meditation. Regular mindfulness meditation workout can useful resource with pressure bargain, emotional well-being, and well-known resilience.

Yoga and Tai Chi are every slight styles of bodily workout that include motion, respiratory strategies, and meditation. These physical video games inspire rest and pressure reduce price even as furthermore improving flexibility, stability, and electricity. Before starting any physical training software program, stroke survivors have to speak with their medical doctor. They may also additionally furthermore discover it useful to paintings with a certified teacher who can modify the recurring to suit their precise necessities and talents.

Social assist and treatment are vital for assisting stroke sufferers deal with the intellectual problems they will revel in while improving. Participating in guide agencies or one-on-one remedy intervals can offer a dialogue board for expressing emotions, converting memories, and getting advice from friends and specialists who are acquainted with the manner of enhancing after a stroke. Counseling and social assist can help with pressure management and emotional health.

There are severa advantages to incorporating those strain discount and rest strategies right right into a stroke survivor's regular normal. Remembering that stroke rehabilitation is a unique and top notch system, it's far vital to alter the ones techniques to house every body's necessities and opportunities. A greater thorough and fruitful stroke rehabilitation method will result from encouraging a holistic approach to restoration that takes underneath interest physical, cognitive, and emotional nicely-being.

STRATEGIES FOR PREVENTING RECURRING STROKES ARE COVERED.

MEDICATION COMMITMENT AND CHANGES IN LIFESTYLE

Effective preventative measures are required for stroke, a awesome motive of mortality and morbidity international, to decrease the threat of repeated strokes. While there are numerous medical remedies available, medicine adherence and way of life adjustments are important in preventing stroke recurrence. To prevent repeated strokes, this article examines the want of medicine adherence and manner of life changes.

Medicine Compliance:

1. Importance of Medication: The risk of subsequent strokes is appreciably reduced through manner of drugs endorsed after a

primary stroke, together with antiplatelet drugs (e.G., aspirin, clopidogrel), anticoagulants (e.G., warfarin, direct oral anticoagulants), statins, and blood stress-reducing medicinal capsules. For lengthy-time period stroke prevention, it's essential to take these tablets as prescribed.

Medication adherence is probably hard for some of reasons, which incorporates the subsequent:

a) Patients might not absolutely recognize the cost of drug adherence or the functionality repercussions of non-adherence.

b) Polypharmacy: The complexity of taking severa particular pills and the bad effects that go with them also can purpose non-adherence.

c) Price: Patients' access to their prescribed medicinal pills may be hampered by charge issues.

d) Forgetting to take tablets or having hassle organizing their schedule: Patients also can additionally neglect to take their medicinal tablets or struggle to set up their remedy routine.

Healthcare practitioners can placed the following 3 thoughts into exercising to decorate treatment adherence:

a) Counseling and training: Giving patients an intensive clarification of the importance of their prescriptions and their blessings facilitates boom adherence.

b) Reduce the huge shape of every day doses or integrate drug treatments into aggregate pills to make medication regimens much less complicated to comply with.

c) Reminder gadgets: Patients can help themselves bear in mind to take their medicinal capsules by using the use of alarms, pill organizers, or cellphone applications.

d) Dealing with monetary boundaries: Looking into charge-powerful picks, like traditional tablets or affected person help packages, can help reduce monetary problems.

Changes in Lifestyle:

1. Healthy Eating: Reducing the hazard of similarly strokes through manner of adopting a balanced weight loss program immoderate in fruits, vegetables, whole grains, lean proteins, and wholesome fats. For people with a data of stroke, it's important to emphasise a low-sodium weight loss plan and limit the consumption of saturated and trans fats.

2. Regular Physical Activity: Regular bodily pastime can enhance cardiovascular health and reduce the risk of stroke recurrence. Swift cycling, swimming, or strolling are a few examples. Additionally, exercise lowers ldl ldl ldl cholesterol, blood pressure, and body weight.

Chapter 10: Management Of Cholesterol And Blood Pressure

Strategies for stopping recurrent strokes include controlling ldl ldl cholesterol and blood stress. A stroke, a essential scientific sickness that develops whilst the mind's blood deliver is reduce off, may be lethal. People who've as quickly as had a stroke are much more likely to enjoy some different one. However, the hazard of recurrent strokes may be considerably reduced via successfully handling blood strain and ldl cholesterol.

Hypertension, sometimes called immoderate blood strain, is one of the essential risk elements for stroke. The blood vessels are strained, so that you can growth the chance of harm and constriction. Uncontrolled immoderate blood pressure can also result in blood clot formation, that could obstruct blood waft to the thoughts and bring about a stroke. Thus, controlling blood pressure is crucial for heading off recurrent strokes.

Changing one's way of life is one of the essential techniques to manipulate blood strain. The DASH (Dietary Approaches to Stop Hypertension) weight loss plan, which prioritizes culmination, greens, whole grains, lean proteins, and coffee-fats dairy merchandise whilst minimizing sodium, saturated fat, and cholesterol, is the type of. Regular exercising is likewise crucial since it lowers blood stress and enhances cardiovascular fitness in preferred. The upkeep of a healthful weight, moderation in alcohol consumption, and abstinence from cigarette use are similarly way of existence modifications which could assist manage blood stress.

Medication can be administered further to lifestyle modifications to govern blood strain. These tablets relax blood vessels, reduce fluid retention, and reduce familiar blood pressure. Examples encompass angiotensin-changing enzyme (ACE) inhibitors, angiotensin receptor blockers (ARBs), diuretics, and calcium channel blockers. People should hold a near eye on their blood strain and abide with the aid of their scientific health practitioner's commands approximately using drugs and dose adjustments.

Another important thing of preventing repeated strokes is handling ldl cholesterol. High cholesterol levels, in particular low-density lipoprotein (LDL) ldl ldl cholesterol, can hasten the onset of atherosclerosis, that could be a disorder marked thru the buildup of plaque in the arteries. A stroke can also prevent cease end result from a ruptured or blocked plaque.

The manage of ldl cholesterol is significantly inspired by way of the use of way of life modifications, much like the management of blood pressure. A coronary heart-healthful food regimen low in ldl cholesterol, trans fat, and saturated fat can assist lower LDL cholesterol levels. Increasing your consumption of end result, greens, whole grains, lean proteins, and healthful fats like the ones in nuts, seeds, and fatty fish is one way to do that. Maintaining specific levels of cholesterol moreover blessings from ordinary workout and weight manipulate.

Medication may be counseled while way of life adjustments by myself are insufficient to govern ldl ldl cholesterol. The most often prescription drugs for decreasing cholesterol are statins. They characteristic through encouraging the removal of LDL ldl ldl cholesterol from the bloodstream and lowering the synthesis of ldl cholesterol inside the liver. In some times, doctors may additionally suggest wonderful tablets which encompass bile acid sequestrants, ldl cholesterol absorption inhibitors, and PCSK9 inhibitors.

To take a look at the efficacy of manner of life adjustments and capsules, ordinary ldl ldl cholesterol tracking is crucial. This regularly entails everyday blood assessments to degree the stages of triglycerides, immoderate-density lipoprotein (HDL) cholesterol, LDL ldl cholesterol, and cutting-edge ldl cholesterol.

Healthcare professionals can adjust the remedy method efficiently based completely in reality on the findings.

Recurrent strokes should be prevented through dealing with blood stress and cholesterol properly. The cornerstone of prevention strategies is way of lifestyles adjustment, which incorporates a nutritious weight loss program, not unusual exercise, weight control, moderate alcohol intake, and abstaining from tobacco products. In addition, tablets may be administered to decrease ldl ldl ldl cholesterol and blood strain. To ensure that those treatments are reducing the threat of recurrent strokes, regular monitoring, and follow-up with healthcare professionals are essential.

CONTROL OF DIABETES AND MONITORING OF BLOOD SUGAR

People who have as quickly as had a stroke run a giant risk of developing recurrent strokes. Effective solutions have to be put into exercising to stop recurrent strokes and decorate lengthy-term consequences. Diabetes mellitus has been determined as a great contributor to the listing of stroke danger elements. To save you recurrent strokes in diabetics, it's far critical to manipulate blood sugar degrees and control diabetes. The courting amongst diabetes and stroke is tested in this newsletter, alongside facet the impact that blood sugar ranges have on stroke hazard and the importance of diabetes control and blood sugar monitoring as preventive techniques.

Diabetes is a metabolic situation marked by using manner of manner of expanded blood sugar tiers added on thru inadequate insulin synthesis or insulin resistance. It has an effect on numerous organ structures and could growth the danger of numerous problems, which includes stroke. Compared to people with out diabetes, humans with diabetes have an progressed hazard of having a stroke. The terrible consequences of continuously high blood sugar levels on blood vessels, significantly the arteries providing the thoughts, are in rate for this elevated danger.

Blood Sugar Levels and Stroke Risk: Elevated blood sugar ranges have a position in the onset of atherosclerosis, a disorder marked with the aid of way of the accumulation of fatty deposits (plaques) inside the walls of the arteries. Vascular stenosis, decreased blood deliver to the mind, and an progressed chance of stroke are all results of atherosclerosis. A stroke is also much more likely to develop due to the fact immoderate blood sugar stages inspire infection, blood clot formation, and harm to the blood vessel lining.

Achieving right diabetes manage is essential for preventing recurrent strokes. Diabetes control as a protection measure. Effective diabetes control is caused through the usage of some essential elements. Maintaining healthy blood sugar degrees in the goal variety suggested thru healthcare professionals is the number one and number one requirement. This regularly consists of pretty a few way of life adjustments, which consist of retaining a wholesome weight, getting ordinary workout, and taking prescribed diabetes medicinal pills, which encompass insulin or oral hypoglycemic stores.

Blood Sugar Monitoring for Stroke Prevention: A key factor of dealing with diabetes is habitual blood sugar monitoring. It allows humans to evaluate their glucose manage and alter their remedy method as vital. Regular blood sugar monitoring is essential for preventing strokes. People who cautiously reveal their blood sugar tiers can spot any changes or irregularities and take right now motion. This preventive method reduces the opportunity of protracted hyperglycemia, which drastically will increase the hazard of stroke.

Collaboration with Healthcare Professionals: It is essential to paintings together with healthcare experts to control diabetes and take a look at blood sugar levels. To optimize remedy regimens and guarantee adherence to advocated techniques, regular checkups and discussions with clinical clinical docs, diabetes educators, and dietitians are important. Healthcare specialists can provide advice on food options, exercising regimens, remedy administration, and one-of-a-kind life-style modifications custom designed to the individual's unique requirements. They also can preserve music of the individual's development, spot possible problems, and provide the proper remedies as required.

Optimal diabetes control and ordinary blood sugar tracking are critical additives of a entire method for stopping recurrent strokes in people with diabetes. The danger of stroke may be considerably decreased through preserving blood sugar stages within the purpose variety and often tracking glycemic control. To create individualized remedy regimens and comply with suggested strategies, humans with diabetes have to art work closely with healthcare carriers. People with diabetes can enhance their desired health and decrease their threat of recurrent strokes via the usage of enforcing the ones preventive steps.

AWARENESS OF WARNING SIGNALS AND SEARCH FOR IMMEDIATE HELP

A stroke is a scientific emergency that must be dealt with right away. The risk of lengthy-time period damage or perhaps dying will growth with the period of time it takes to are seeking out for medical interest following a stroke. For a stroke recovery to be effective, the warning signals of a stroke ought to be identified and early help sought. In this publish, we'll have a take a look at the stroke caution symptoms and talk approximately what to do if they'll be noticed.

Strokes can show up unexpectedly, therefore it's vital to pick out the signs and symptoms as quick as possible. The acronym "FAST," which stands for: let you bear in thoughts the maximum ordinary stroke warning symptoms and signs and symptoms.

Face drooping: The face may additionally droop or get numb on one difficulty. Check to look if the individual's smile is choppy thru asking them to smile.

One arm can also additionally moreover begin to revel in numb or prone. Ask them to elevate every fingers and watch to peer if one arm falls.

Speech problems: Slurred or difficult-to-recognize speech is viable. To take a look at for any speech irregularities, ask the character to copy a brief sentence.

It is vital to call emergency services proper away and get medical assist if any of those signs are present.

Additional stroke caution symptoms and signs and symptoms can embody:

A sudden, horrible headache that is in contrast to any other headache you've got got ever had may be a signal of a stroke, particularly if high-quality signs and symptoms are present.

Vision troubles: Sudden double vision, blurred or impaired vision in a single or every eyes, is probably a sign of a stroke.

Dizziness and absence of balance: During a stroke, a person also can experience a sudden lack of stability, coordination, or dizziness.

Numbness or vulnerable point: On one side of the body especially, numbness or weakness within the face, arm, or leg may be a warning signal.

Seeking Immediate Help: It's critical to do so proper away if you or a person you understand is displaying symptoms and signs and symptoms of a stroke. When you phrase the caution signs and symptoms and signs and symptoms and signs, follow the ones instructions:

Dial the emergency amount proper away (in the US, it would be 911) and describe the signs you're experiencing. Declare your suspicion of getting a stroke in order that the proper movement may be taken.

If you are with someone who's showing stroke signs and symptoms, stay with the beneficial resource in their thing till assist arrives. Keep them calm and reassure them.

If you may, write down the time at the identical time as the symptoms and signs first appeared. For deciding on the remarkable route of remedy, this facts might be important.

Do not forget about the symptoms; despite the fact that they seem to head away or get higher, you want to nonetheless see a medical doctor. TIAs, usually called "mini-strokes," can stand up earlier than a primary stroke and need to not be left out.

Avoid riding your self or the person that is having stroke symptoms to the medical institution: It is usually counseled toward using your self or the patient to the medical institution. While at the manner, emergency clinical services can offer the favored attention and transportation.

Recovery from a stroke relies upon on being privy to the signs and signs and getting care proper away. When it includes stroke treatment, time is the essential factor because short scientific hobby can reduce mind harm and increase the danger of a entire recuperation. We can save you deaths and decrease the extended-term results of strokes by means of using manner of being aware about the warning signs and acting short.

Chapter 11: The Many Movements Of The Shoulder Joint

Lateral rotation **Medial rotation**

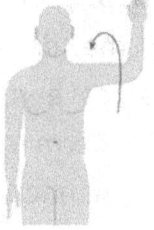 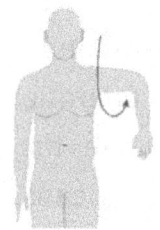

If you have got got were given the benefit of having a person with you, positioned your non-affected hand on their shoulder blade (scapula) as they perform most of these moves. You will sense the remarkable angles and motions the scapula movements in because the arm is moved.

In the illustrations, you can moreover see the pleasant posture of the spine and shoulder girdle as those moves are being finished.

POSTURE IS ESSENTIAL

Communication a number of the spinal wire to the mind and to the limbs may be compromised if the backbone or spinal cord is in terrible posture.

An important tip whilst appearing your physical remedy and/or schooling (exercising) on posture, balance, status and/or walking talents is to hold your eyes looking in advance. Your body follows your eyeballs. If you appearance or face down, the body will try to study, as established within the bad posture photographs. It will keep you in terrible posture.

Proper posture of the backbone bones

and determination muscle groups is crucial.

The spine is made of

7 cervical vertebrae,

12 thoracic vertebrae,

five lumbar vertebrae.

The sacrum is 5 vertebrae fused collectively.

At the lowest of the sacrum is the coccyx, this is known as the tail bone (Not demonstrated in illustrations)

The manner I bear in thoughts the range of vertebrae is with the aid of a announcing my university professor taught me.

"We consume breakfast at 7:00, lunch at 12:00 and dinner at 5:00."

The Nerves

The example of nerves above does now not encompass all of the nerves which is probably involved in moving the arms. I percentage this to expose in which the nerves originate from the spinal twine and then via the higher vertebrae for arm, hand, and finger movements. This is the the the front view.

The nerves are very complicated, and I received't be going into high-quality intensity of these nerves. I will fine be sharing some essential records to the nerves on this arm instance.

Brachial plexus is a plexus of nerves. Plexus is form of a network. I moreover see it as branches. Many branches that increase out to specific locations. These branches of nerves make bigger from the spinal wire, via the cervicoaxillary canal inside the neck, over the primary rib, and into the armpit. It is accountable for the motor innervation of all the muscle businesses of the arms, fingers, and palms.

Pectoral nerve is responsible for the pectoralis maximum crucial and minor—the chest muscle tissues.

Musculocutaneous nerve: The musculocutaneous nerve innervates the 3 muscle mass of the anterior compartment of the arm: the coracobrachialis, biceps brachii, and brachialis. It is likewise answerable for cutaneous innervation of the lateral forearm.

Radial Nerve: The radial nerve is a peripheral nerve that offers motor and sensory characteristic to the arm. It turns on the medial and lateral heads of the triceps and 12 muscle agencies placed within the wrist and fingers. This nerve provides cutaneous sensation to posterior quantities of the thumb, index finger, middle finger, and the lateral 1/2 of the ring finger. An damage or limited or lack of conversation with this nerve can bring about the disability to increase the arm, wrist, and arms. Cutaneous sensation is the felling of warm, cold, contact, strain and pain through the pores and skin.

Thoracodorsal nerve is likewise referred to as the middle subscapular nerve or the prolonged subscapular nerve. It activates the latissimus dorsi (lats) muscle. This also method this nerve plays a feature in activating the moves of extending, adducting, and internal rotation of the shoulder. You'll test extra at the latissimus dorsi muscle later in this ebook. There is likewise more in-intensity understanding in my ebook The Power of Your Spine, How Back Strength and Posture Pilots the Entire Body.

Ulnar Nerve is the most vital nerve in the body this is unprotected with the aid of using muscle groups and bone. When you bang your arm and enjoy an ordinary sensation (tingling/numbness), it's far the ulnar nerve being hit. It is often referred to as "hitting the humorous bone." This nerve is one of the number one nerves inside the arm. This nerve starts offevolved at the neck and travels via the shoulder and down the arm into the wrist, palms, and arms. It is a part of the brachial plexus nerve department.

Although the ulna nerve passes via the forearm, it's miles simplest chargeable for a number of the forearm movements. Its number one feature is to provide nerve characteristic to the hand. It is also referred to as the "musician's nerve" due to the reality it's miles chargeable for the fantastic movements of the fingers.

Median Nerve turns on the flexor muscle tissues of the forearm and hand. This nerve moreover turns on the flexion, abduction, opposition, and extension of the thumb and distinct additives of the arms.

POSTURAL MUSCLES

Before we glide immediately to the various muscle groups that assist pass the arm, allow's communicate about the psoas. If you have got take a look at my first 4 books, a number of what I'll proportion about the psoas and the postural muscle groups can also sound acquainted. The psoas is a without a doubt vital muscle positioned inside the center of the body. It lies deep under the transverse belly muscle. It is a deep back muscle. It is the simplest spinal muscle that right now attaches to the legs. The psoas muscle is the extraordinary muscle inside the again that crosses over the hips and attaches on the the the front of the frame. It attaches on the final thoracic vertebrae and to four of the five lumbar vertebrae and on the femur, the pinnacle thigh bone. It is also the bridge the various hips and the returned. Often it's miles called the iliopsoas. This is while the psoas and the iliacus muscle organizations are being grouped collectively.

If the stomach muscle mass are susceptible, the psoas and awesome muscle groups will try to do their way. If the psoas is short, susceptible and/or tight, it is going to be tough to preserve the body in an upright function with the shoulders stacked over the hips. There will also be more of a mission for a stroke survivor if the psoas has spasticity in any of its fibers. Spasticity does now not only show up inside the arm and legs. It can take vicinity in any muscle within the frame. For example, if there can be spasticity in a single or some of the multifidus or spinal rotatores, it can make it extra tough to art work on posture, balance, and stabilization of the backbone and frame. This is every different purpose to maintain operating on strengthening the center and postural muscle groups. See my one-of-a-kind e-book Stroke Recovery What Now? When Physical Therapy Ends, But Your Recovery Continues. It has a monetary disaster on middle and backbone muscle groups and a financial disaster on bodily games.

Multifidus

The multifidus is a small however effective muscle. It is the principle stabilizing muscle of the spine. This muscle takes strain off the vertebral discs in order that the frame weight may be dispensed at some stage in the spine. If that is vulnerable, you could moreover have weakness inside the low decrease back. The multifidus starts offevolved offevolved offevolved to activate in advance than the body moves to guard the backbone. It is part of the stabilizing device in the body. The multifidus is likewise one of the muscular tissues in the spine that extends, abducts, adducts, and rotates the spine. In order to advantage better balance, this muscle need to be strong. Performing numerous sports activities combining with the Swiss ball, balance disc, balance pad and BOSU® ball will assist benefit a more potent multifidus. Better posture ends in higher stability. See my books, Tipping Toward Balance or Stroke Recovery What Now? For carrying sports on balance and stabilization.

To help this sound less hard, whilst we bend over from the spine (rounding the spine), that is called spinal flexion. When we're pulling the spine from flexed function lower decrease back as plenty as being upright, this movement is referred to as spinal extension, additionally referred to as Axial Extension. Flexion is while a muscle brings joints together. Extension is bringing the 2 joints farther aside. For example, at the same time as we flex our arm to expose our arm muscle tissue (the bicep) as in acting a bicep curl workout, that is flexion. As you expand the arm lower lower again out right away, this is extension.

The small muscle businesses close to the vertebrae want to be activated harmoniously. These muscle mass are postural muscular tissues. Exercising on an unstable floor, together with the Swiss ball, stability disc, balance pad and the BOSU® ball, stimulates the imperative annoying device, which might be the mind and the spinal wire. It strengthens muscle mass and ligaments, similarly to activating and strengthening all of the small muscle tissues along the spinal column.

The multifidus muscle, transverse stomach muscle, diaphragm, and the pelvic floor muscle tissue are all on the same neuromuscular loop. This means it's miles super if a majority of these muscle corporations are functioning properly; each wants to perform its interest for my part and as a group. Stated a piece more complicated, it manner a sequential segmental neuromuscular stimulation with closed loop remarks. If the transverse muscle is prone, the pelvic ground, the multifidus, and the diaphragm can't benefit right power to perform their jobs in a wholesome, functioning frame.

Often stroke survivors want to decorate and correct their posture. Even for seniors and others with balance and stabilization problems, gaining robust postural muscle businesses is essential. Proper posture should be strengthened to assist the opportunity stabilizing muscular tissues to keep the frame strongly upright definitely so it could acquire a posture wherein the shoulders are stacked over the hips. If the top is upright and balanced over the shoulders, we've higher balance. The balance in the pelvis and hips should be made so that the decrease limbs and joints can benefit electricity, characteristic in alignment, and carry out properly for secure actions.

In the example above, the proper aspect shows sections best for reading. They aren't interested by their entire attachments inside the route of the backbone.

The Transversospinalis organization consists of:

The rotators, interspinales, and intertransversarii.

These muscle businesses are vital for offering proprioception remarks many of the thoughts, again, and complete body.

Rotators - The mission of those muscle tissues is to boom the spine and rotation to the opportunity facet. It moves with proprioception, bringing stability while the frame is in motion. They extend the backbone and rotation to the alternative aspect. This organization of muscle organizations has lots to do with proprioception, in particular the rotators and the interspinales. The interspinales has masses to do with the comments the various lower once more and brain and from the mind to the decrease lower back. They are the inner most (deeper than the multifidus) and have the maximum medial layer of spinal fascia. "Medial" approach it's miles the nearest to the center of the body.

Interspinales – Segmental extension. This muscle brings numerous proprioception for the once more, stability and stability of the spine and body in movement. Segmental extension of the spine way arching the again.

Intertransversarii – Small segmental movement and lateral flexion of the spine.

They are small muscle groups which can be on every elements of the backbone.

The Interspinales and Intertransversarii muscle groups circulate and stabilize the backbone. They furthermore play a large position in frame consciousness and proprioception.

Therefore, it's so critical to bolster the center and determination from the interior out. The frame communicates from motion and actions beginning deep inside the spine. This is why after I teach customers to regain their stabilization and cognitive talents such balance, spatial popularity and proprioception, I begin with smooth but extraordinarily powerful sporting activities like recognition on balance discs, stability pads, and/or BOSU® Balls to rebuild the ones muscle businesses and their herbal communication to the thoughts and again.

Quadratus Lumborum

The quadratus lumborum (as you may see interior the example above) is attached from the lumbar vertebrae and rib 12 to the crest of the ilium. It stabilizes the pelvis (hip girdle) even as strolling, and laterally flexes the spine. It performs lateral flexion. It has 3 layers of fibers that go along with the float in 3 particular hints. The quadratus lumborum can cause plenty of ache if you are having problems or a awful damage. When this muscle is satisfactory activated (or in spasticity) on one side, the trunk is bent inside the route of that path.

The instance of the quadratus lumborum (QT) on the proper shows that if one aspect of the QT is shorter than the possibility element, it can hike up the pelvis/hips. This will have an impact at the entire body. It can have an effect on shoulder joint and arm movements.

When someone sits with their hips off to 1 facet, that is what the deep muscle groups of the spine will do. The Psoas and others as well.

For instance, if someone is attempting to have a look at to stroll once more, and that they spend a extraordinary deal time sitting with the muscle tissues in this function, once they go to stand or stroll, they may now not have the strength, stability, and muscle connection to regain the capacity at their splendid. These illustrations are also some other seen to expose the energy of the spine muscle groups and a right posture.

Here is a quick phase on a number of the center muscles. I want to additionally are seeking for advice from them due to the fact the postural muscle tissues and the stabilizing device. If you need to observe extra approximately center and resolution electricity and carrying sports to enhance them, see my other books at www.Amazon.Com/author/tracymarkley.Com or www.Tracymarkley.Com

Chapter 12: Transverse Abdominal Muscle

The transverse muscle is the inner maximum of the belly muscle tissue. Without this muscle being sturdy, the multifidus spine muscle cannot be sturdy. The transverse muscle's critical function is to stabilize the decrease lower again and pelvis in advance than motion. It is the inner most belly muscle, wrapping around the frame to behave like a corset. It enables stabilize the hips and pelvic. When engaged, it furthermore pulls the belly in and affords guide to the thoracolumbar fascia, and it's far the stabilizer of the shoulder girdle, the pinnacle, neck, pelvis, and lower extremities.

For mother and father which is probably seeking out to correct posture or are in rehabilitation to discover ways to stand and stroll once more or someone who has rounded shoulders and terrible posture, it is essential to decorate this muscle. It need to be reinforced to assist the opposite stabilizing muscle mass to keep the body strongly upright in order that it could achieve a posture in which the shoulders are stacked over the hips. If the head is upright and balanced over the shoulders, we've got better balance. The balance inside the pelvis and hips need to be made surely so the lower limbs and joints can advantage strength, feature in alignment, and carry out properly for secure movements.

Before we pass ahead to every other muscle, I choice it's far turning into clearer to you without a doubt how muscle groups artwork together to help extraordinary muscle organizations inside the frame perform their jobs.

The pelvic floor muscle agencies paintings as stabilizers of the stomach and pelvic organs. The pelvic ground muscle tissues and the gluteus (buttock) muscle tissues are made to paintings and circulate in opposite commands. One need to be capable of have interaction the pelvic floor with out engaging the gluteus muscular tissues if you want to collect ultimate middle power. These muscle businesses have to be separated within the thoughts and worried system for ordinary frame functioning. This plays a feature in preventing all over again problems. The transverse muscle have to be strong for the pelvic ground to end up robust and function nicely considering they are at the same neuromuscular loop.

Reminders

In each one in each of my books, I share this within the anatomy section:

The transverse belly muscle, the multifidus muscle, diaphragm, and the pelvic ground muscular tissues are all on the identical neuromuscular loop. This technique it is amazing if these kinds of muscle businesses are functioning well; each desires to carry out its way in my view and as a team. If the transverse muscle is inclined, the pelvic floor, the multifidus, and the diaphragm can not benefit proper strength to carry out their jobs in a healthful, functioning body.

Transverse

Multifidus

Pelvic Floor Muscles

See my ebook Stroke Recovery What Now? When Physical Therapy Ends, But Your Recovery Continues, for extra special statistics on center and posture muscle tissue and wearing sports activities to enhance the center and stabilizer muscle groups.

The Other Abdominal Muscles

The Transverse Abdominals had been referred to earlier inside the ebook. Now allow's have a look at the possibility 3 stomach muscle mass.

Rectus Abdominus

This is the maximum superficial belly muscle. This is the muscle that creates the "six p.C." appearance. It attaches on the the front of the ribs five through 7 and to the pubis. It flexes and adducts abducts and adducts the backbone. It lets in the lean of the pelvis and the curvature of the low backbone. It moreover adducts the ribs inflicting exhalation. Often whilst humans simply do stomach crunches and no real sensible schooling of the abs and center, this muscle can get tight, inclusive of or causing lower again pain.

Internal Oblique

The phrase oblique, consistent with the Oxford Dictionary, technique neither parallel nor a right mind-set to a line, however slanting at an mind-set. Both the Internal and External Oblique muscle fibers run on an mind-set.

The Internal Oblique is on the lateral (side) detail of the trunk. It attaches at ribs 10 thru 12 and to the crest of the ilium (pelvic bone). It adducts the ribs, causing exhalation. It moreover flexes, abducts and adducts, and rotates the backbone.

External Oblique

The External Oblique attaches from rib five through 12 and to the crest of the ilium. It adducts the ribs, causing exhalation and flexes, rotates, adducts and abducts the backbone.

If the deep spine muscle tissue which you examine about in advance in this e-book are prone and not acting their task well, those outer muscle organizations will pull extra hard at the spine, that would bring about damage and malfunction. It can be very important to enhance the body from the internal out, much like a toddler develops. This is a key to stability, backbone and lower returned care, proprioception, stabilization, and protection of the spine. It is also the important thing to building all of the backbone and center muscle companies to their satisfactory power so all the muscle companies can interest on great the assignment they had been made to do. This additionally leaves the frame plenty a good deal less fatigued.

The Glutes

In the preceding example, you may see the huge glute muscle tissues and the smaller muscle corporations which is probably under. The large glute muscle tissues make bigger the femur, that's the backswing of the leg in walking. It moreover rotates the femur outward. The smaller organization of muscles artwork together to rotate the femur outward. The femur is the huge better thigh bone. In the instance on the proper, you could see how the Latissimus Dorsi muscle groups meet the thoracolumbar fascia and paintings with the possibility issue glute muscle tissues. See my different books for additonal on this.

We have a gluteus maximus, medius, and minimus. The gluteus maximus extends and rotates outward even as the gluteus medius and minimus abducts and rotates the femur inward.

If the backbone and again muscular tissues are willing and there is terrible posture, the hips and pelvic will no longer be robust and stable sufficient to permit these muscle agencies and precise muscle companies just like the piriformis and the opposite hip rotator muscle companies you spot in this situation to artwork well. This leaves the spine and again muscle tissues to try to help within the ones muscle mass' jobs, leaving the frame searching for to feature and circulate out of balance, inflicting pain, weak spot, and harm inside the lower lower back as well as hips, knees, and ankles. Posture is important!

There are many muscle groups that participate inside the actions of the arm. For example, muscular tissues that hook up with the scapula (shoulder blade) will play a thing in arm movement. There are severa muscle businesses that hook up with the humerus (top arm bone) and the scapula. This way any muscle that permits flow the scapula may additionally even assist the motion of the arm because the scapula actions in masses of arm movements. Even the biceps and triceps join at one element to the scapula.

Teres Major attaches at the scapula and the humerus. It extends, adducts and rotates the humerus inward. The humerus is the better arm bone.

The Teres Minor is one of the 4 rotator cuff muscle groups. It attaches at the scapula and to the humerus. It extends and rotates the humerus outward. The scapula is the shoulder blade.

Serratus Anterior attaches on the scapula and to ribs 1 via 9, and it rotates the scapula outward.

Reminders

Scapula is the shoulder blade.

Ulna is one of the bones inside the forearm. The distinct one is the radius.

Humerus is the higher arm bone.

Rhomboid Major attaches on the scapula and the backbone at the cervical vertebra (neck). It rotates inward and adducts the scapula.

Rhomboid Minor attaches scapula and the spine. It rotates inward and adducts the scapula.

Reminders

If the spine is in right posture, the scapula may be capable of circulate more glaringly and freely. This will assist the arm to regain its movements.

The Rotator Cuff Muscles

There are four muscle groups that make up what is called the "rotator cuff."

These four muscle tissue art work together as a set to maintain the shoulder girdle well in region just so the shoulder joint can move freely and properly. These four muscle agencies are the Supraspinatus, Infraspinatus, Teres Minor, and Subscapularis. They art work as a collection, however also have their movements that they carry out on their own. Maintaining horrible posture at the same time as the use of the shoulder joint in everyday sports, together with exercise on this horrific form in all the one-of-a-type modalities, can cause an harm. It isn't always unusual to pay attention clients say they have got a "rotator cuff harm" and now not understand which muscle or ligament it's far. Many in truth count on it is a cuff and do not understand that there are genuinely four muscle corporations creating the so-referred to as "cuff."

Supraspinatus attaches on the scapula and the humerus.

It abducts the humerus.

Infraspinatus attaches on the scapula and the humerus. It extends and rotates the humerus outward.

Teres Minor attaches on the scapula and the humerus. It extends and rotates the humerus outward.

Subscapularis attaches on the scapula and the humerus. It adducts and rotates the humerus inward.

As you can see, all four muscles connect at the scapula and the humerus. However, every of those rotator cuff muscles attaches at one-of-a-kind areas of the scapula and at specific regions of the humerus. To maintain it simple, I did not list the correct component of attachment.

Reminders

Scapula is the Shoulder blade.

Humerus is the higher arm bone.

Adduct manner including a part of the body decrease returned towards the midline of the body.

Abduction technique transferring part of the body further from the midline of the body.

Rotation outward way rotating a part of the body faraway from the midline of the body.

Rotation inward manner rotating a part of the frame once more toward the midline of the body.

Muscles that join on the scapula and humerus must be activated to regain arm motion once more. This manner acting bodily sports activities and movement remedy that skip the scapula.

Keep the shoulder down at the identical time as sitting, popularity, and workout.

When you commonly have your shoulders raised up into your ears, it places the shoulder girdle and joint in a negative functioning movement. This will now not top notch purpose injuries but placed a pull at the fascia that is going thru the body and backbone.

It additionally continues the trapezius and a few neck muscle mass in persevered flexion. This will purpose pain and disorder in movements and can result in extra again, hip, and pelvic pain in masses of people. The stroke survivors I artwork with regularly have a partial or entire shoulder dislocation, and once I placed it back in location, and that they preserve their shoulder down (which means they prevent flexing the muscular tissues that boom the shoulders to the ear), the shoulder can then heal and get again in its proper characteristic. It also can assist release hip pain and tightness. A partial dislocation is likewise known as a subluxation.

Trapezius Muscle

The Trapezius muscle mass are in 3 sections— the superior, medial, and inferior. Superior manner above. Medial method center. Inferior manner decrease.

The Superior Trapezius attaches to the scapula, the cranium, and the vertebrae. It abducts the scapula.

The Medial trapezius attaches horizontally from the scapula to the vertebrae. It abducts and inwardly rotates the scapula.

The Inferior trapezius attaches to the scapula and the vertebrae below. It abducts and inwardly rotates the scapula.

Trapezius adducts the scapula, tilts the chin, attracts returned acromion and rotates the scapula.

Reminders

Scapula is the shoulder blade.

Humerus is the top arm bone.

Vertebrae are small bones that form the backbone/backbone. They every have numerous projections for articulation and muscle attachment. They each have a hollow thru which the spinal cord passes.

Performing carrying sports that assist circulate the scapula will help gain mobility inside the scapula (shoulder blades), which ends up in extra mobility and interest of the humerus.

Don't forget approximately the Rhomboids.

Stay in pinnacle posture as you perform your sports sports/bodily therapy.

Latissimus Dorsi

Often Referred to because of the truth the "Lats"

The Latissimus Doris adducts, extends, and medially rotates the humerus. It attaches at the hip and lower lower returned and into the thoracolumbar fascia and to the humerus (the better arm bone).

The thoracolumbar fascia allows the lower once more muscle groups and allows them acquire the capacity to move the body. It is made from robust fibers and allows channel forces of motion as the again muscle tissue settlement and loosen up. The nerves to those muscle businesses additionally skip thru this fascia. This fascia is going deep to the spine and is made from 3 layers. It is essential for contralateral motions like taking walks. It works with the latissimus dorsi (lats) to coil the center of the frame.

When the thoracolumbar fascia is supported, it permits all of the muscle companies that connect with it to feature better. These muscles embody the gluteus maximus, latissimus dorsi, trapezius, erector backbone, quadratus lumborum, psoas, transverse, and internal obliques. It lets in bridge the muscular tissues of the decrease again to the muscle corporations of the stomach wall. This fascia lets in integrate the movements of the higher body with the decrease body. Nerves from seven unique muscle groups inside the middle run through the thoracolumbar fascia.

See extra about the power of the spine muscle mass and the thoracolumbar fascia in my e-book The Power of Your Spine, How Back Strength and Posture Pilots the Entire Body.

Serratus Anterior is mounted on the scapula and to ribs 1 thru nine, and it rotates the scapula outward.

Chapter 13: The Chest Muscles

Pectoralis Major attaches at the sternum, the clavicle, and the humerus. It flexes, adducts, and rotates the humerus inward.

Pectoralis Minor attaches at the scapula and to ribs three, four and five. It adducts and rotates the scapula outward.

Deltoids

The Shoulder

The Anterior head of the Deltoid attaches at the clavicle and the humerus.

The clavicle is the collar bone. It flexes, abducts, and rotates the humerus inward.

Medial head of the Deltoid attaches at the scapula and the humerus. It abducts the humerus.

Posterior head of the Deltoid attaches at the backbone of the scapula and the humerus. It extends, abducts, and rotates the humerus outward.

Sternocleidomastoid attaches to the mastoid method, sternum (breastbone) and clavicle (collar bone). It flexes, rotates, abducts and adducts the backbone.

Reminders

Scapula is the Shoulder blade.

Humerus is the better arm bone.

Clavicle is the collar bone.

Anterior is in the direction of the the front.

Medial is within the middle.

Posterior is toward the decrease again.

Arms, Hands and Finger Muscles

There are many muscle corporations within the route of the fingers, hands, and fingers. To assist maintain this e-book smooth, I simplest wrote out targeted muscle attachments and movements for a number of the muscle tissues tested inside the illustrations.

Triceps: "Tri" method 3. The Triceps muscle has three heads.

Medial head of the triceps brachii attaches from the humerus to the ulna.

It extends the forearm.

Lateral head of the triceps brachii attaches from the humerus to the ulna

It extends the forearm.

Long head of the triceps brachii attaches from the scapula to the ulna.

It extends the forearm. (Straightens the elbow/arm) Extending the forearm is honestly unbending the elbow and straightening the arm.

The Triceps extends the forearm.

Flexion is while a muscle brings joints collectively. Extension is bringing the two joints farther apart.

Biceps: "Bi" way . The Biceps muscle has two heads

Biceps brachii prolonged head attaches at the scapula and radius.

It flexes the forearm. (Bends the elbow)

Biceps brachii brief head attaches at the humerus, scapula, and radius.

It flexes the humerus. (Bends the elbow)

Coracobrachialis: This muscle is a joint muscle. It attaches on the humerus and the the the front of the shoulder joint at the scapula. It flexes the humerus.

Biceps Brachii: This muscle is a joint muscle. It attaches on the radius and the the front of the shoulder joint on the scapula. It flexes the humerus.

The radius, also called the radial bone, is the bigger bone of the 2 forearm bones. The forearm bones are the radius and the ulna.

Pronator quadratus attaches to the radius and ulna. It allows the radius to go over the ulna. It moreover rotates the forearm inward.

Flexor pollicis longus attaches to the radius and the thumb. It flexes the thumb.

Flexor digitorum profundus is attached at the ulna to the 4 fingers (not the thumb). It flexes the palms (now not the thumb).

Did you realize the word "profundus" manner deep?

The following hand illustrations display some of the severa muscle agencies that are within the hand. I display those to help it make revel in as to why seeking to flow into the palms and fingers in all one-of-a-kind angles and moves will help carry again actions.

Reminders

The wrist flexes (bending/curling up) and extends (starting), moves component to side, and may rotate in spherical motions.

The arms flex (bending/curling up), extend (setting out/straightening), moves factor to element, and might rotate in round motions.

As I actually have shared in advance than, I am no longer a bodily therapist. I am a fitness expert who sought superior education to help me in assisting stroke survivors the top notch I can once they have finished their physical treatment. In the following pages you'll discover a combination of wearing sports and pointers that would help for your restoration.

This first workout is an average hand exercising that many survivors are given.

I attempt to remind my clients to open their hands as big as they're able to among each finger to thumb touch. No depend what level you are at in this exercise collection, attempt to start with the hand as tremendous open as you can get and finish as huge as you may.

When you stand on a BOSU® ball or a balance disc together along side your hand for your element and perform these bodily sports activities, the critical tense gadget is inspired greater, therefore growing better improvement in the movements and recovery.

Try specific angles and actions at the same time as workout the palms to assist deliver the hand and arms decrease again to fuller functioning.

Spread the palms.

Open the hand, close to the hand.

Make circles with the wrist and hands.

Touch every finger one at a time to the thumb. While doing this, try to open the hand decrease returned up among every thumb contact. Work on the whole extension of the fingers and hand.

If possible, and whilst solid, stand on BOSU© ball, balance pad, or stability disc and maintain onto a few component for safety with the non-affected hand whilst strolling on the affected hand and arm.

If secure and in a function, you may additionally take a seat down on a balance ball even as doing hand bodily sports activities.

Try beginning with movements within the rhomboids and top back earlier than doing hand bodily video games. This will set off the muscle groups and nerves in the path of the spinal twine first earlier than transferring right down to the hand bodily sports.

Pick up marbles, pins, or small devices from one pile or cup/bowl and go with the flow to some other cup/bowl.

In this workout above, begin by means of way of pulling the shoulder blades collectively, then have the arm observe via thru bringing the elbows again, then improve the fingers over again and repeat. This may be accomplished like inside the picture or with a band, as you may see in other photographs.

Bounce balls.

Try to fold towels or cloths.

While sitting at a table, you can use any of those system or some exceptional you could have.

You can use what items you've got got got in your private home, however the ones are the machine within the photograph I actually have:

Balance disc

Form curler

Dish towel

Cup

Small items – paper clips, massive clips a glue stick.

Therapy putty

Therapy Eggs

A big yoga/Pilates ball and a small weighted ball

A wood round bar/stick

A finger/difficult treatment tool

Balance disc for sensation and protective as a tool.

A ball, bar, and foam roller to roll inside and out together along with your fingers and fingers.

Small devices, collectively with paper clips, paper clamps, treatment putty, treatment eggs, a small weighted ball, and a therapy device used to help unfold the hands and different carrying activities. I will share some sporting occasions right right right here. Continue with unique wearing events out of your therapist if they're running.

Roll out the froth roller flat with one hand and/or fingers.

Stand roller up and rotate it in circular motions with the palms/hands.

Roll the ball far from you, then bring it lower lower lower back inside the route of you.

Rotate the ball problem to facet to assist with kind of motion with the shoulder and wrist.

Remember, in all the arm sporting activities, whether you are sitting or fame, stay in proper posture. Keep those shoulders in right positing.

Roll a bar to and fro. With all of the rolling out sporting activities, you may use both palms and one hand.

Play with the squishy treatment eggs. Try to close the hand and open the hand. Do the finger workout you saw in advance in the e-book, via the use of on the lookout for to contact every finger one after the alternative to the egg. Keep gambling along with your gear and maintain the fingers and hands continuously trying to make all the precise movements they will make.

The fingers can skip surely into this tool or maintain the tool towards the fingertips. Open and near the hand. Play and check.

Use treatment putty and wonderful remedy belongings which have been endorsed or given to you through your therapist. The putty may be unfold out on a desk, and you can have your hands unfold it open and play with it. All those device encompass instructions, similarly to a therapist can be able to educate you extra.

Continue the wearing sports that your therapist has given you as you add in different sporting occasions.

When succesful, paintings on making the distinct shoulder movements formerly shared in the illustrations on pages 1 and multiple of this e-book.

One facet of the stability disc has a bumpy element. By urgent the hands on this bumpy element it may assist stimulate the nerves in the hands and palms. You can workout and try to circulate your arms in unique angles and movements on the disc, by way of searching for to hold every finger in my opinion. You can preserve it amongst your fingers and squeeze. You can rotate the disc round and do different finger and hands actions in this selection. You can hold it like a steerage wheel of a automobile and make the movements as if you are turning the steerage wheel. (Not shown in photographs)

Rotate the disc side to element to assist with style of movement with the shoulder and wrist.

In the photo above, I am the use of the Anchor Point Training® band that is attached to the ceiling in my studio. I am urgent down with without delay palms and slowly controlling the motion once more up. This works the lats, traps, triceps, and shoulders. It is also strolling balance, stability, and the center. Your body have to trap up on the pull of the band with the resource of no longer letting it pull you ahead or circulate backward. With all of the wearing sports that require every fingers, you can have the non-stroke affected hand maintain the effected aspect so it is able to comply with the moves if it's miles not able to transport however on its personal.

Remember to hold posture the extraordinary feasible and interact your middle at the identical time as doing all of your arm and hand sports activities activities.

Try to set off those specific movements to help deliver all actions yet again.

Do them with the unaffected component first. Feel what it looks as if. Do it together with your eyes open, see it, and visualize it. If viable, do the actions together together together with your eyes closed additionally. Stay centered and try to feel and visualize it. Then at the same time as you figure at the stroke-affected thing, try and experience and visualize it doing what the alternative hand did. In fact, do this with all sports for the arm, palms, and arms. And consider, protection first!

Hold on with the non-affected hand and exercising the stroke-affected hand.

Be fine to maintain onto a sturdy object which includes a bar secured to a wall.

Stand in a right posture with the abs engaged.

Chapter 14: The Non-Affected Hand

The sporting activities shared on this ebook can be completed sitting, status, fame on BOSU® ball, stability disc, stability pad, kneeling on a BOSU® ball, sitting on a ball, or sitting in a chair. Ensure your protection first. Then even as equipped and steady, you can strive the extra advanced techniques.

As the center and postural muscular tissues advantage energy to preserve your body upright within the proper posture with balance and stabilization, the arm moves can gain more recuperation.

Kneel in a proper posture with the abs engaged.

Sit with proper posture with abs engaged.

When you engage your abs, DO NOT squeeze your butt muscle agencies.

Many wearing sports may be with the ones exceptional positional options being shared in this ebook.

Your therapist has with a chunk of good fortune given you some remedy carrying activities to do. Keep doing them. Incorporate them into posture, balance, and middle sporting sports each time viable. This additionally enables the mind multitask once more. These duties bring stability and stabilization due to the fact the arm and fingers pass. This can take time, staying strength, and repetitive safe workout.

Currently, most of you've got were given already been thru treatment, or you are though receiving treatment. Either manner, proper right right here are a few bodily activities that could assist you in getting movement once more thru your arm, hand, and palms. As I said in advance in this ebook, I am not a bodily therapist. I am a fitness teacher who often receives clients who have finished their physical treatment and do not realize what else they could do or how a excellent deal similarly their recovery can bypass. Stroke survivor's healing does now not prevent whilst bodily therapy ends.

You might also additionally quality be capable of do some of the physical sports in this ebook as well as a number of what your therapist has proven you. Do the wearing sports that you could do and are capable of do correctly.

When possible, begin with center and postural carrying occasions.

Standing on a balance pad, disc, BOSU® ball, or kneeling on BOSU® ball is a tremendous way to heat up the center and postural muscle mass. This additionally strengthens those muscle corporations and stimulates the vital worried gadget. It additionally enables teach the frame to multitask over again and permits rebuild spatial focus and brief reaction time. This builds stability and balance. These are extraordinary heat-up and physical sports activities to do for fall prevention.

Move the shoulders and the shoulder blades.

Get the muscles and nerves deep on the backbone activated by status on surely considered one of the stableness system or sitting on a ball (while organized).

Do the higher decrease back and lat muscle wearing occasions.

This exercising above may be finished at the ground or on a BOSU® ball.

Keep your abs engaged, thigh bones (better leg) right away up and down. Do not permit them to attitude out proper proper right into a plank function. Hinge at your hips because the ball rolls out, then press fingers/hands firmly into the ball as it pushes your frame once more upright in correct posture. This strengthens center, lats, triceps and shoulders, and mobility.

While performing exercising on the BOSU® ball, it moreover works balance, legs, glutes, and stability. Exercise Tips Continued

www.ingramcontent.com/pod-product-compliance
Lightning Source LLC
Chambersburg PA
CBHW070759040426
42333CB00060B/1212